Secrets of Health and Joy in All Seasons

A Practical Guide with the Wisdom of
Traditional Chinese Medicine

By Su Liqing

SCPG

Text by Su Liqing
Translation by Bleanor Bouttell at BESTEASY
Cover design by Shi Hanlin
Interior design by Wang Wei

Assistant editor: Qiu Yan
Editor: Cao Yue

ISBN: 978-1-63288-007-9

Address any comments about *Secrets of Health and Joy in All Seasons* to:

SCPG
401 Broadway, Ste.1000
New York, NY 10013
USA

or

Shanghai Press and Publishing Development Co., Ltd.
Floor 5, No. 390 Fuzhou Road, Shanghai, China (200001)
Email: sppd@sppdbook.com

Printed in China by Shanghai Donnelley Printing Co., Ltd.

1   3   5   7   9   10   8   6   4   2

Contents

Foreword

Many have heard the saying that "prevention is better than cure." More and more, people are choosing to pay close attention to their general health, aging and longevity, and prioritizing their health care and quality of life. However, the majority of people lack systematic knowledge of how to care for their health. This book collects healthcare knowledge from the world of traditional Chinese medicine, and outlines a different perspective on health care, in order to help a wide variety of needs.

The book's design has three main tenets. First, it is systematic and comprehensive. It outlines methods of health care according to the four seasons of spring, summer, autumn, and winter, systematically introducing health care tips from the perspectives of prevention, exercise, entertainment, diet, lifestyle, emotional health, and physiotherapy. Second, this book uses popular, easy-to-read language, expressing complex medical concepts in a way that is accessible to everyone. Third, the contents of this book are convenient and practical. Healthcare methods are introduced in a memorable and concise way, so that readers can easily apply what they have learned to their lives.

This book helps you live in tune with the year's four-season rhythm, allowing you to make health-preserving habits part of your daily life. This is your shortcut to year-round physical and mental health.

Chapter One
Spring

In the theory of seasons, spring always marks new beginnings. The return of spring means more sunshine warming and brightening the earth, and a thriving natural world, full of life. Breathing in the fresh spring air, full of the smell of new flowers and shoots of grass, and listening to the chirps of insects and birds, is one of life's purest joys. However, just as the earth has a night and a day, there are two sides to every season. Spring is one of the best seasons of the year, but also a season in which disease recurrence is common. For this reason, we must take good care of our health in spring, using this time period to lay a good foundation for a healthy full year.

Spring is a time for the ascending and dredging of *yang qi*, (the positive, *yang*, form of *qi*, a Chinese medicine concept denoting pure life energy) and the budding of all things. Humans are part of the natural world, and our metabolisms respond to the *yang qi* of spring by becoming stronger. Consequently, many generations of healthcare experts have long supported the idea that spring is a time for nourishing positive energy, or *yang qi*. In practical terms, this means we should choose appropriate forms of exercise to nourish our physical fitness. One might take morning and evening walks on grass trails, for example, or go shadow boxing (Tai Chi), sword dancing, hiking, or on retreats to the countryside. Being amongst natural scenery such as mountains and rivers, appreciating the beauty of blooming flowers, and finding one's way to high-up spots to admire faraway views are all practical ways to improve both physical and mental health.

According to the Five Elements Theory fundamental to traditional Chinese medicine, the liver is associated with the element of wood, and ascends in spring as a tree thrives in spring, resisting restraint or depression. Because of this, looking after your liver is of great importance during spring. The key to nourishing the liver is to regulate emotions, that is, to control your seven emotions: joy, anger, worry, thoughtfulness, sadness, fear and shock. If you think or worry too much, it can affect the flow of *qi* from your liver, disrupting the ascending and descending movement of *qi* in your body. This in turn upsets the balance and function of *yin* and *yang* energy, or *yin qi* and *yang qi*, in your body, influencing your blood and viscera, resulting in a cluster of diseases. In short, the key to health in spring in traditional Chinese medicine is maintaining *yang* energy and protecting the liver.

1. Prevention in Spring

Air temperatures and weather patterns in spring can be unpredictable, with both warm and cold air circulating. The instability of the climate can cause problems for the vulnerable, such as individuals who have pollen allergies, seasonal allergies (e.g., allergic rhinitis), or suffer from asthma. Springtime is often windy. Wind pathogen is an important concept in Chinese medicine, and is cited as a main cause of disease in spring. Wind pathogens may cause various infectious and epidemic diseases, such as colds, diphtheria, scarlet fever, rubella, pink eye, measles, meningitis, chickenpox, tonsillitis, pneumonia and so on. Traditional Chinese medicine is a holistic practice, and believes that the human body coordinates with the rhythms of nature. In spring, therefore, the human liver responds to the rising *yang qi* of spring, with liver *qi* and liver fire ascending. This powerful liver *yang* can lead to hypertension, dizziness, hepatitis and other health problems. This surging *yang qi* in the liver can also influence your mood and mental state, resulting in a sort of "high" or mania. Individuals suffering from schizophrenia, mania or other mental disorders may be prone to anger, agitation, argumentativeness, and other non-optimal states.

Springtime Lethargy

Do you ever feel a little lazy when the weather finally begins to warm in spring? Do you ever find that you feel lethargic, even if you've had a good night's sleep? This is what we call springtime lethargy.

Springtime lethargy is not a disease, but a temporary physiological phenomenon of the human body adjusting to the changes of the seasons and air temperature. In winter, in order to adapt to the cold, protect the body's warmth and prevent energy loss, the microvessels on the skin contract. This maintains the body's physiological base temperature, and increases the activation of the central nervous system, so the mind is relatively clear. In spring, however, when the temperature is more moderate, the skin and the body's microvessels are in a state of relaxation and blood flow is slower. There is a greater supply of blood to the body's surface, while the supply of blood flowing into the brain is slightly reduced. The central nervous system is less active and stimulated, resulting in the sleepy "springtime lethargy" phenomenon.

It should be noted here that some forms of "springtime lethargy" are symptoms of diseases. For example, depressive symptoms before the onset of psychosis; low fever and lethargy in the early stages of hepatitis; lethargy related to diabetes or heart disease. Some people also found that patients with hypertension, especially elderly patients, are lethargic and yawn frequently in spring, which may be a sign of oncoming stroke. As a result, anyone with the above symptoms is recommended to go for a full medical checkup.

It is normal to feel drowsy in the spring, but if an individual shows signs of excessive sleepiness, it indicates an underlying disease or a health issue. For optimal health in spring, follow the natural laws of spring by doing three things:

Have a regular and consistent sleep schedule. Traditional Chinese medicine believes that regular sleep restores the spirit and one's vital energy, *qi*. Without a regular sleep schedule, one's mood and mindset can easily become disrupted and chaotic. It also results in a decline in the adaptability to the environment, which leads to various diseases.

Yang qi ascends in spring, and the generation of this positive *yang* energy is closely related to sleep. When we are awake, our *yang qi* is at the surface. When we are asleep, it moves inside. When conducted properly, a slight reduction of sleep time is conducive to an ascension of *yang qi*. Having too much sleep does not relieve fatigue, and will in fact increase sleepiness, because the main reason for springtime lethargy is not a lack of sleep but rather a lack of stimulation of the nervous system and cells. Excessive sleep can make the body's *yang qi* stagnate, thus blunting the functions of the cerebral cortex.

Regulating the body and mind helps disperse stagnated liver *qi*. Spring as a season is connected with the liver organ. If the liver is functioning normally, the movement of *qi* around the body will be smooth, helping prevent disease. The liver is a master of filtration, and has the function of dredging and filtering all the body's *qi*, blood and clear fluid. The physiological expression of liver is *qi* ascension, and if it is functioning normally, *qi*, blood and clear fluid will be flowing smoothly. When the flow of one's blood and *qi* energy is unblocked, clear *yang* ascends, rising all the way through the body to the brain and nourishing it, effectively eliminating lethargy. In contrast, if liver *qi* stagnates or is blocked somehow, then the *qi* movement cannot occur unimpeded. Clear *yang* is blocked and the brain cannot function at its optimum state, resulting in springtime lethargy.

Traditional Chinese medicine believes that the liver disperses *qi* and does not like to be blocked. To maintain normal liver function, one must support the liver's physiological characteristics. Therefore, in spring, you should keep your mood relaxed and avoid anger, and depression that harms the liver. Physical exercise such as walking outside or practicing Tai Chi can not only relax your muscles, but also help your *yang* energy ascend, unblock your blood vessels and invigorate your spirit. In this way, your blood flow will be smooth, your frame of mind will be relaxed, and you will have plenty of energy.

Ensure your food combines the Five Flavors. "*Yang* is the key to health preservation in March." If *yang qi* is flowing freely in the body, and the movement of *qi* is properly regulated, your mind will be clear. If *yang qi* is deficient for any reason and the *qi* movement is out of balance, fatigue will easily occur. *Yang qi* is born in the spring. The best way to respond to this is to support the ascension of *yang qi* in your physical body any way you can. In terms of diet, traditional Chinese medicine recommends adhering to the principle of "eating to nourish *yang* in spring and summer," a concept dating all the way back to *The Yellow Emperor's Classic of Medicine*. In practical terms, this means eating more pungent and sweet foods, such as onions, garlic, coriander, and so on. These kinds of foods help replenish *yang qi*, enriching the positive energy of the human body and promoting its ascension.

Healthy people can easily combat springtime lethargy with the above methods, while those who are in sub-optimal health conditions, such as with imbalanced *yin-yang*, disharmony of *qi* and blood, or weakness in organ function, may find a longer duration of springtime lethargy that is not easy to correct. Such patients should engage in systematic health recovery at their earliest convenience.

Dermatitis

In spring, the temperature fluctuates, and the air is full of pollen. At this time, the skin is prone to acne due to the overproduction of sebum. Spring is the most sensitive season for the skin. Spring dermatitis is a photosensitive skin disease. Its main cause is having a skin allergy to the sun's ultraviolet rays. Of the four seasons of the year, ultraviolet rays are at their lowest levels during winter. When spring comes, however, there is a sudden rise in ultraviolet rays, which can be hard for some people to adapt to. Exposure to strong ultraviolet rays can cause skin damage and dermatitis (skin inflammation).

Spring is also, however, a peak season for outdoor activity and travel. Forgetting to apply sunscreen can induce or aggravate dermatitis. In addition, improper use of seasonal skin care products, such as using winter creams during the spring, can easily cause blotching and other allergic reactions.

Rubella

Rubella is an acute airborne infectious disease caused by the rubella virus, mainly seen in spring. The main symptoms are malaise, fever, inflamed upper respiratory tract, swollen lymph nodes behind the ear and the occipital region, and light red papules rapidly spreading across the whole body, which is extremely itchy and unpleasant. Generally, the papules fade rapidly in two to three days without leaving any trace. Rubella has little impact on the general population, but for pregnant women, infection with the rubella virus can cause fetal deformities, premature birth, or even death, and thus proper prevention is crucial.

Hay Fever

In spring, many people experience sneezing, runny or stuffy noses, headaches, eye watering and related allergic symptoms. Rather than a cold, these can also be hay fever. Hay fever is a collective name for pollen allergies, an allergic reaction caused by plant pollen and pollen mites. As flowers pollinate during spring, the amount of pollen floating in the air increases sharply, and it can easily enter the body as you breathe. This can cause allergic reactions in the respiratory tract, eyes and skin. In addition to the above symptoms, some sufferers also experience severe itching in the upper palate, external ear canals, nose, eyes and elsewhere. Symptoms may also include localized or generalized hives, recurrent facial dermatitis, and itching. In severe cases, sufferers may experience chest tightness, difficulty breathing or asthma. Spring is the flowering season for many trees, and tree pollen is a common allergen. People with allergic constitutions are easily affected by pollen when outside. Therefore, corresponding measures should be taken, such as:

① Stay away from allergens. Avoid likely allergen hotspots such as botanical gardens and other places where there are a lot of flowers and trees. Avoid outdoor trips in places where plants are flowering and pollinating, and try to minimize the presence of house plants.

② Take preventive medicine. In the weeks before the arrival of the pollinating period, use sodium cromoglicate which has a strong preventive effect on hay fever.

③ If an allergic reaction develops, you should leave the environment you are in and take antihistamines. Any medicine, such as Astemizole, should only be used under the guidance of doctors to avoid side effects.

Colds

People catch colds in all seasons. Colds, also sometimes called upper respiratory tract infections, have the main symptoms of nasal congestion, a runny nose, sneezing, a dry or sore throat, hoarseness, cough, sputum and so on. Although spring colds are common, if they are not treated properly or in time, they can lead to many complications, such as sinusitis, stomatitis, laryngitis, otitis media, lymphadenitis, pneumonia, and bronchitis.

Flu is another common infectious disease, which can occur all year round, but has a higher incidence rate in spring and winter. How to avoid colds and flu:

① Ensure a good flow of fresh air into indoor spaces.

② Fumigate a room with peppermint essential oil or rice vinegar to purify the air.

③ Try to eat less greasy, sweet foods, such as fish and red meat, and eat more foods that help prevent respiratory tract infections, such as carrots.

④ When treating a cold, utilize pungent and cool-natured drugs to resolve superficies syndrome and clear away heat and toxins. In the early stages of a cold, use Ban Lan Gen (isatis root extract) and associated medicines. Those with severe symptoms should seek medical attention.

⑤ Massage treatments can also be used to prevent and treat colds, such as Zusanli point acupressure. The Zusanli acupoint is located 3 cun (four finger widths) down the outer Xiyan acupoint and about one finger length from the outside of the tibia. During a massage, press heavily on the Zusanli acupoint on the same side with the thumb, and place the other four fingers

Body Length Measurement

Using Thumb Length	Using Middle-Finger Length	Using Four Fingers Closed Together
The width of the patient's thumb joint is 1 cun. This is applicable for locating the acupoint on four limbs with vertical cun.	With the patient's middle sections of the bent middle finger as measurement, the distance between two inner crease tips is taken as 1 cun, which is mostly applicable for locating acupoints on four limbs with vertical cun and on the back with horizontal cun.	With the index finger, middle finger, ring finger, and small finger of the patient stretched straight and closed, measure at the level of the large knuckle (the second joint) of the middle finger. The width of the four fingers is 3 cun.

1 cun

1 cun

3 cun

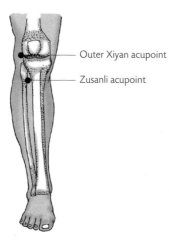

Outer Xiyan acupoint

Zusanli acupoint

behind the lower leg against it, increasing the pressure until there is some local soreness. Then, press and knead on the same acupoint on the other leg.

Cardiovascular Disease

The climate in spring gradually changes from cold to warm, but this is only a general trend. The climate in spring is the most volatile of all four seasons, and in fact, one feature of spring is that the cold can surprise you when it returns after a spell of warmth. This can give the springtime chill a more powerful effect on health than the chill of winter. Cold is often an inducing factor for cardiovascular diseases. Therefore, with the continuous change between cold and warm weather in spring, there is a high incidence of cardiovascular disease. The onset of coronary heart disease, hypertension, myocardial infarction and other diseases in spring is very common. If treatment is delayed for any reason, it can lead to serious consequences.

Allergic Rhinitis

Spring is a painful season for many patients with allergic rhinitis. This is because the temperature fluctuates and the air is filled with pollen, which is the main allergen causing rhinitis in spring. In addition, dust mites, household chemicals, irritant fumes and protein-rich foods can also cause allergic reactions in the nose. Allergic rhinitis can significantly affect one's daily life and work, and also may induce a variety of complications if improperly treated. The most common complication is bronchial asthma, but other complications include sinusitis, otitis media, allergic rhinitis. It is therefore important not to ignore allergic rhinitis and treat them in a timely manner.

Hair Loss

Dry weather and a surge of ultraviolet rays from the sun make spring the season most associated with hair loss. In spring, the scalp is dry, and the hair is fragile, dry and prone to break, especially in March and April.

If the amount of hair loss per day is 50 to 100 strands, don't worry too much. This is normal for the human body. More than this, however, is excessive and should not be ignored. Having a poor lifestyle, which can mean being in a stressful environment, eating an overly greasy diet, living a sedentary lifestyle, having an irregular sleep cycle, excessive smoking or alcohol consumption can all result in male hair loss, especially in the spring. For females, in addition to stress levels and sleep deprivation, hair loss is also related to hormone levels in the body.

In spring, the hair should be washed with running water every morning, and combed through gently with a wide tooth comb. In addition, it is important to eat more protein-rich foods. Supplementing your diet with extra vitamin A can also reduce hair loss.

Other Spring Diseases

After the beginning of spring, people start to wear fewer layers and enjoy the warmth. However, experts warn that people should beware of eight types of spring diseases.

Pneumonia: The beginning of spring is the season of a high incidence of lower respiratory tract infections, especially in children. The incidence rate is more than four times higher than that in summer. Before infection with pneumonia, people often suffer from upper respiratory tract infections, which start with a sudden chill, and then develop into a fever, coughing and difficulty breathing. This can be accompanied by nausea, vomiting, and muscle soreness. It's a dry cough at first and then accompanied by sputum with pus or blood in it.

Prevention: Fumigate rooms with rice vinegar, and take isatis root extract to prevent the spread of disease. Ensure a regular flow of fresh air to your working and living environments. Make sure you wear appropriate clothing for the weather, and exercise regularly. If you experience a fever, coughing or other symptoms, seek medical attention.

Measles: Measles usually occurs in winter and spring. The disease is transmitted through respiratory droplets. People who have never had measles and have not been vaccinated against it are generally susceptible. Children aged six months to five years have the highest incidence rate. Measles is an acute respiratory infectious disease caused by the measles virus. It is characterized by a fever, cough, runny nose, bloodshot eyes, and a rash around the mouth that may spread across the body. It is often complicated by pneumonia and can endanger the lives of infants and young children.

Prevention: Children should avoid crowded places. If infected, individuals should be isolated and treated as early as possible. Children with measles should be isolated until five days after rash onset.

Mumps: A common infection seen frequently between winter and spring. Mumps is an infectious disease caused by the mumps virus. It can be transmitted through contact, droplets and several other ways. The main symptoms of mumps are a central swelling under the earlobe, accompanied by obvious pain or tenderness; difficulty in opening the mouth; fever; decreased appetite. The general incubation period for mumps is two to three weeks. Swellings are often seen on one side first, and then the other side, with pain and a hot sensation.

Prevention: Utilize the mumps vaccine. Use nasal or oral sprays (that is, atomization treatment. Nasal spray equipment is relatively simple, generally a handheld spray bottle used for applying for liquid medicine).

Myocardial infarction: Sufferers with myocardial infarction often experience angina for more than three to five minutes or even half an hour before onset. Sufferers may also experience chest tightness, difficulty breathing, and fatigue. In spring and winter, the temperature fluctuates, making it easy to get sick. Prevention: Keep warm and avoid the cold. Ensure work and rest are properly balanced, and avoid excessive fatigue and long-distance travel. Keep your mood relaxed. Avoid overeating and exercising after a meal. Eat less high-fat foods. Those who are overweight should consider broader dietary changes.

Hepatitis: Viral hepatitis A and E, which are enteric infectious diseases caused by the hepatitis A and E viruses respectively, are clinically characterized by fever, nausea, vomiting, liver pain, jaundice and liver dysfunction.

Prevention: Do not eat raw or half-cooked seafood. Develop the personal hygiene habit of washing your hands before meals and after using the toilet.

Pink eye: Pink eye is an acute infectious eye disease caused by bacteria or viruses. It is most likely to occur in the spring and summer, and outbreaks are common in schools and other places where people gather closely together. Pink eye is mainly spread through physical contact.

Prevention: The best way to prevent pink eye infection is to have good hygiene. This means washing one's hands frequently, and never rubbing your eyes with your hands. When pink eye is prevalent, it is advisable to avoid swimming or bathing in public pools and shared locker rooms. If someone in your home has been infected with pink eye, other people who are not sick should brew and drink a preventive tea of 10 grams of mulberry leaves and 20 grams of chrysanthemum.

2. Exercise for Spring

In spring, people should engage in exercise that suits their physical condition. This not only replenishes the *yang qi* consumed by the cold weather in winter, but also creates clear fluids of *yin* nature ready for the coming summer months. It is best to avoid high-intensity exercise in spring, as excessive exercise can actually have adverse effects on the body's *yang qi* and growth. The most appropriate forms of spring exercise are moderate and done outdoors, such as jogging, or practicing Tai Chi or *qigong*. The air outdoors is full of negative oxygen ions, which are a good nutrient for promoting the growth of human bones. Although they can't be seen or touched, they are "floating" around constantly in the air, and are very useful for preventing children's rickets and osteoporosis in the elderly.

Considerations for Springtime Exercise

Don't bare too much skin. Fog and high winds are common in spring, so when exercising outdoors, it is important to limit contact with cold and damp air in order to prevent joint pain. Do not exercise in places where the air is thick with dust particles, and learn to inhale through your nose and exhale through your mouth to keep your airways clear.

Make sure you warm up your joints before any exercise. Swing your arms, kick your legs, and turn at the waist to make sure all muscles and joints of the body are active and relaxed before you engage in any strenuous exercise.

Exercise should be full-body. As well as stretching your limbs, also consider movements that engage and stretch your back, abdominals and chest. During or after exercise, do not lie down on the grass. This can easily cause lower back pain or problems in the joints. The maximum heart rate during springtime exercise should be 130–150 bpm.

Always ensure you are properly dressed to avoid catching a cold. If you, like most people, sweat as you exercise, take care not to spend too long in wet clothes. These can easily give you a chill, and the effect is worsened by windy weather.

Avoid exercising too early in the morning in spring. This is because in early spring, particularly in February, the temperature is very low in the mornings, and such cold air can be bad for your immune system. If you exercise outside very early in the morning, you make yourself very vulnerable to "wind pathogens." In mild cases, this results in a cold, but in severe cases, exposure to cold wind pathogens can cause joint pain, stomachache, and even facial paralysis, angina and multiple other problems. Environmental monitoring data also shows that the air is typically cleanest in summer and autumn, while air pollution is more severe in the first two months of winter and spring. Six am is a peak time for air pollution. The more intensely you exercise, the more air you inhale, and thus the more harmful pollution particles you breathe in.

Walking

Walking outdoors is a great form of easy health care, especially during spring as the weather warms and flowers begin to appear. After a long day of work, taking a walk is also a good way to dispel fatigue. One well-known secret of longevity is setting aside a certain amount of time every day to take a walk, especially in spring when the climate is comfortable and there are plenty of things for your eyes to appreciate. Both of these are conducive to good health.

How fast you walk can be easily adjusted to whatever is comfortable, and the same goes for the duration. Ideally, a walk should be a consistent effort and result in a very light sweat. The elderly should walk slowly and steadily, aiming for a pace of perhaps 60 to 70 steps per minute. This simple act can stabilize the mood, eliminate fatigue, and also have the effect of strengthening the stomach and helping digestion. Young, middle-aged and elderly people with a high level of fitness can incorporate faster walking, which is classed as about 120 steps per minute. This faster pace is still easy and pleasant, and consistently walking this way helps lift your spirits, improve your brain function and increase the strength of your lower limbs. When walking, you might also incorporate your arms, adding movements such as rubbing your hands, massaging your chest and abdomen, slightly beating your back, or patting your whole body, to encourage blood flow and generate *yang qi*.

Nourishing the Liver and Eyes

In spring, *qi* coming from the liver is of crucial importance.
The liver is connected to the eyes via meridians, and as such,
anything that looks after the liver also helps nourish the eyes.
The eyes are prone to fatigue during spring, and are vulnerable
to infection, especially if you spend long stretches of time sitting
down or looking at papers or screens. The following methods are
some ways to properly look after your eyes:

Eye care: While working on something or looking at
a screen, close your eyes and rest for a while every 40 to 50
minutes to relax your eyes.

Eye pressure points: Massage the acupoints around the eyes
to promote blood circulation and improve the supply of fluid and
nutrients to the eyes.

Finding a view: Relax your eyes by finding a pleasant view
to look at. Watching spring scenery in the distance helps adjust
your retinal cells and relieve visual fatigue.

It should be emphasized that in spring, to nourish both
the liver and eyes, we should go to sleep earlier and generally
make sure we have a healthy sleep schedule. Spring is a common
time for flare-ups of conjunctivitis, so it is also a good idea to
pay special attention to eye hygiene. Do not rub your eyes with
unwashed hands or dirty towels, napkins and so on. This goes a
long way to preventing eye diseases.

Combing Head Massage

Why do healthcare practitioners place so much importance on
combing one's head and hair in the spring? In spring, *yang qi*
ascends and dredges across the globe, rising upwards towards
the sky. The *yang qi* in the human body also adapts to the
changes in the spring climate. Rising early and performing a
combing head massage is one way to help your *yang qi* rise. The
head is the locus of the five human senses, as well as the central
nervous system. Regular massage can improve blood circulation
to the head, as well as nourish the hair, making it shiny and

rich in color. Regular massages can also help improve vision and hearing, relieve headaches, and prevent high blood pressure and stroke risk, amongst other benefits.

Below is one outline for a combing head massage that incorporates *qigong* techniques:

① Stand upright with your feet shoulder-width apart, knees slightly bent, chest pulled back, shoulders sunk and hands dropped. Keep your eyes open and look straight ahead. Consciously relax, eliminate all distractions, and concentrate on the "elixir field"—an energy center acupoint—found 3 cun below the navel.

② Maintain a state of quiet, and slowly lift your hands, gently pressing your palms to your forehead. Gently rub down your nose all the way to your jaw, then go up the back of your head and neck, gently rubbing over your entire head before returning to your forehead. This movement should be done 36 times. Start out softly the first time, and then gradually increase the pressure.

③ Bend your fingers, but keep them separate, so that each hand creates a cupped shape, then starting from the hairline of your forehead, press your fingers over the top of your head, all the way over until you get to the back of your neck. Gently grasp at your scalp as you move your fingers. Then, move your hands away from the front and rear midline of your head gradually, still gently grasping at the scalp as you go until you reach the upper ears. This movement should be done 36 times. Start out softly the first time, and then gradually increase the pressure.

④ With the same cupped hand shape, starting from the upper hairline of the opposite ear, massage across the top of the head to the upper part of the other ear. Then, using the line between the two ears through the top of the head as the center, move your left hand forward and the right hand backward, gradually separating them while gently grasping at the scalp until you have thoroughly massaged the front and back hairlines. Do this 36 times, starting lightly and gradually increasing pressure.

⑤ Lay your palms on your face, and starting from the forehead, rub down to the lower jaw, then turn to the back of your head and neck, and rub from the top of your head to your forehead. This movement should be done 36 times. Use light pressure to begin with, and then gradually increase it.

This combing head massage is an organic combination of both hair combing and cranial massage. It encourages the entire body to relax, and increases concentration, helping you breathe evenly and move more fluidly. The pressure should be gentle at first and increase gradually. Remember not to press too hard to cause pain or rush it.

Morning Stretches

Stretching on spring mornings is a very good idea. After a full night's sleep, the human body is soft and a little slack, with both *qi* and blood circulating slowly. This is why you always feel lethargic and a little weak when you first wake up. Stretching out your limbs, waist and abdomen first thing in the morning exerts your muscles, and when doing it with deep breathing, it is highly effective at brushing off the heaviness of sleep and promoting *qi* and blood circulation. Stretching helps unblock the meridians and joints, invigorate the spirit to help get rid of tiredness, activate your muscles and thus boost your strength. According to traditional Chinese medicine, "blood pools in the liver when one lies flat, and flows through the meridians when one moves." Stretches help stimulate strong blood circulation, feeding the muscles and joints of the whole body and keeping them active and alert. The liver is also switched on by these stretches, which is in line with the principle of nourishing the liver in spring.

Strengthening the Bones and Kidneys

Spring is also an ideal time to strengthen bones. Traditional Chinese medicine believes that the kidneys are inextricably linked to the bones, and that they are what generates bone marrow. In order to strengthen your bones, you must therefore focus on strengthening the kidneys. Abdominal and waist exercise help with this. The moves below are useful to learn for kidney care.

Rubbing the waist with both hands: Rubbing at your waist with both hands helps disperse the belt channel, strengthening the whole waist area and kidneys within. The waist is where the "belt channel" (a channel of meridians around the waist) lies, and the back of the waist on both sides of the spine is where the kidneys are located. The kidneys like warmth and do not do well in the cold. Regular massage helps keep the kidneys warm, increasing the flow of *yang qi* and blood to them. The specific method is: first rub your hands together to make them warm, then press the waist tightly, pause for a moment, and then rub down to the Changqiang acupoint (the midpoint of the line between the end of the tailbone and the anus). This should be done 50 to 100 times, once in the morning and once in the evening.

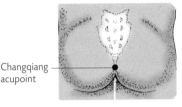

Changqiang acupoint

Lower abdomen massage: Traditional Chinese medicine believes that the kidneys and the bladder are very closely related. The *qi* transformation function of the bladder depends on the rise and fall of kidney *qi*. Kidney *qi* helps the bladder to transform *qi* and clear fluid in the body. Therefore, health care for the bladder also plays an indirect role in protecting the kidneys. The bladder is located in the lower abdomen. One specific massage method for the bladder is as follows: overlap your palms, and place them in the center of the lower abdomen. Press down, and then rotate, first clockwise 20 times, and then counterclockwise 20 times. Push the bottom of the palm of your hand down, from the center of the lower abdomen to the upper edge of the pubic bone, and repeat continuously for three minutes. Massaging the bladder in this way can strengthen the kidneys.

Lightly beating the waist and abdomen: You may have observed some elderly people using their hands to lightly punch the back of their waist, without even thinking about why they do it. Although few can say why they do it, many say it makes them feel more comfortable. What is the reason behind this? In fact, this is also a kind of health massage for the kidneys. It is recommended, therefore, for the elderly to often engage in this light punching technique. When doing this, first brace your legs around shoulder width apart. Legs should be slightly bent, and your arms should hang easily at your sides with hands half clenched. Turn your waist, first to the left, and then to the right. As you do this, start to swing your arms naturally back and forth with the left and right rotation of the waist. Use the momentum of your swinging arms to gently knock the back of your waist, and lower abdomen, one after the other. How hard the impact is can be easily adjusted. This movement should be done around 30 times.

3. Leisure in Spring

Spring is a great time for leisure activities. As birds sing and flowers start to appear outside, there is plenty of opportunity for getting out and moving around in a way that enlivens the body and senses. This helps stimulate the body's *qi* and blood flow, helping nourish the mind and body.

Spring Walks

In winter, the body's thermoregulation functions and the functions of internal organs can drop to a certain extent. After this season of rest and inactivity, the body's muscles and ligaments have often atrophied slightly and are less able to contract. Going out on spring walks in the fresh scenery not only exercises the body, but also cultivates the spirit. Especially in the countryside, the air is fresh this time of year. Flowers and leaves are brightly colored, and there is often the sound of birdsong. These surroundings are very good for your state of mind, and so walking in spring is a great way to promote health.

Flying Kites

Being outdoors, you might also want to consider bringing a kite to fly. This engages the eyes, and can help prevent myopia. Since many plants sprout in the spring, just getting outside and exposing yourself to fresh green colors can be of great benefit to vision, helping relax the eyes.

In the modern age, it is extremely common for people to look at a computer screen or books for long stretches of time. This can easily lead to chronic visual fatigue, increasing the probability of suffering from eye diseases, and accelerating eye-area aging. Thus, it is important to adjust your routine to look after your eyes. The human eye is easily irritated by ultraviolet rays. Rays of white light and red light can also cause strong irritation. Indoor lighting, especially from computers, game consoles and television screens, can easily damage the retina. Looking intently at anything for too long can easily cause tension in the ciliary muscles of the eyes, which not only causes tiredness, but may also cause myopia. As well as being relaxing to the body and mind, outdoor kite flying has particular use in that it helps prevent myopia. It does this by encouraging people to focus their gaze on the far distance, helping to naturally adjust the eye muscles and help them relax and rest. The most common movement patterns of the human eye are looking down at something close by, and looking up at something further away. Finding ways to focus on faraway things is a way to vary the types of movements the eye performs, helping protect overall eyesight and reduce eye fatigue.

Kite flying is also a whole-body exercise that utilizes all the muscles of the body. As an activity, it involves running, holding onto strings and controlling movements with the hands, engaging several different muscle groups and joints.

When the kite rises into the sky, the pull from the wind can be quite powerful. Flying kites, therefore, acts as a resistance exercise, building strength in the arms, waist and back, as well as improving stability in the foot and tibia joints. It can also improve your reaction time. Walking outdoors in the spring, holding a kite in your hands and watching it dance in the wind, is an effective way to lift one's mood. This in turn promotes overall physical and mental health and will aid the recovery of chronic diseases.

Middle-aged and elderly people should pay attention to neck protection when flying kites, and take care not to spend too long leaning backward and looking up. Take frequent breaks for the best results. Kite flying is best done in groups of two or three people. Choose a wide, open space rather than anywhere near a lake or river, and avoid places with high-voltage power lines to avoid accidents.

Using Chinese Hand Therapy Balls

There are many ways to exercise using these handheld therapy balls, and people often group together these exercises under the umbrella term "iron ball exercises." Spring is not the best time for intense exercise, but utilizing these therapy balls is a perfect form of moderate exercise. There are four main benefits of turning these therapy balls over and over in your hands: ① It strengthens blood circulation; ② It builds physical strength; ③ It helps certain brain functions; ④ It can help combat high blood pressure.

Growing Flowers

As well as being nice to look at, flowers also contain substances that purify the air. They help sterilize and disinfect their surroundings, as well as emit pleasant fragrances. When flower fragrances, also called aromatic or essential oils, come into contact with the olfactory cells in the nose, they are immediately transmitted to the cerebral cortex through the olfactory nerve.

This is what creates a refreshing and pleasant reaction in the blood and nervous system. Research shows that different flowers produce different oils. Radish flowers, pumpkin flowers and lily flowers, for example, emit an oil that can treat diabetes. Geranium flower oils can calm the nerves, and aid sleep and brain function. The oil of cardamom flowers can combat stomach diseases, and the styrax flower oil is very effective at reducing high blood pressure and treating coronary heart disease. Research has also found that some plants (such as asparagus fern, cactus, begonia, geranium, etc.) also secrete phytocidin, an antibacterial. The oils of other flowers and plants can repel flies, moths and mosquitoes. Therefore, in spring, why not spend some time playing in the garden? Growing your own flowers will ensure you spend time in close contact with these nourishing plants, with the happy side effect of filling your home with pleasant fragrances.

Of course, there are some things to remember:

① When growing flowers indoors, make sure you have the correct indoor conditions to actually do so; do not overload the room with too many plants. If the windowsill is too full of flowers and plants, it can block the sunlight, which people also need for their health.

② Be aware that some plant and flower oils may give some individuals headaches, or cause asthmatic reactions. Some people are also allergic to pollen. In these cases, flowers should be immediately moved outside or replaced. Some flowers, such as geranium, calendula and primrose, should not be touched by hand to avoid allergic dermatitis or eczema.

4. What to Eat in Spring

Traditional Chinese medicine believes that food is medicine, and as such attaches great importance to putting the right nutrients in your body. Thousands of years of accumulated knowledge have resulted in the passing down of many highly effective medicinal foods, which is a unique feature of Chinese medicine. Spring is the season of rising *yang qi*, so people should adapt to this by regulating *yang qi* through their diet.

Foods to Eat and Foods to Avoid

In spring, *yang qi* ascends and dredges, and the human metabolism begins to flourish. At this time, your diet should include pungent, sweet and warm foods, while sour, astringent foods should be avoided. As a rule of thumb, your food should be light and tasty, and greasy, cold foods should be avoided. Pungent and sweet foods help nourish natural spring *yang* energy, while warm foods help protect existing *yang*. These include foods such as onions, coriander, leeks, jujubes, peanuts, and so on; however, this does not include extremely hot foods, such as ginseng.

The underlying principle of this springtime nutrition is the even reinforcing of the liver and spleen. The liver is the most important organ in spring, because its physiological characteristics reflect that of springtime trees. If the liver is not functioning properly for any reason, this will lead to disorders in the circulation of *qi* and blood around the body, causing a ripple effect of problems throughout the body. The sour flavor strengthens the liver, and the liver is hyperactive in spring. When you ingest excessive sourness in the spring, this can cause excessive liver *qi*, which then affects the spleen. The spleen is closely related to the stomach. A weakened spleen hinders digestion and the absorption of food. Sweet foods, on the other hand, nourish spleen *qi* when ingested, which then helps nourish the liver. In spring, therefore, one should eat fewer sour foods and more sweet foods. This helps nourish the liver and spleen, which is of great benefit to disease prevention and overall health. Grains (such as glutinous rice, black rice, sorghum, millet, oats), fruits and vegetables (such as sword beans, pumpkins, lentils, red dates, longans, walnuts, chestnuts, etc.), and meat and fish (such as beef, pork belly, perch, etc.) are all prime options for sweet and warm foods. These foods are extremely rich in nutrients, and give the liver and spleen what they need to thrive.

It is also a good idea in spring to eat more fresh foods and vegetables rich in vitamin B. Modern diet science shows that a vitamin B deficiency is closely related to springtime lethargy. To ensure you are getting enough vitamin B, eat vegetables like carrots, cauliflower, cabbage, and bell peppers regularly and often. Cold, cool or greasy foods can easily damage spleen *yang*, so try to eat them as little as possible.

Seasonal Vegetables

Spinach: Spinach can nourish blood and *yin* energy (*yin* energy being the negative opposite of *yang* energy), and can effectively combat high blood pressure, headaches, dizziness, diabetic symptoms and anemia, which are often caused by insufficient liver *yin* in spring. However, spinach also contains a high number of oxalic acid, which hinder the body's absorption of calcium. Thus, it is best to first cook spinach in boiling water, and fry it before consuming it. Because infants and young children especially have an urgent need for calcium, and some also suffer from tuberculosis, osteomalacia (soft bones), kidney stones, diarrhea and so on, it is best for them to avoid eating too much spinach.

Shepherd's purse: Shepherd's purse contains oxalic acid, tartaric acid, malic acid, fumaric acid and other active ingredients. These have the effect of eliminating dampness and soothing the spleen, as well as aiding blood coagulation and brightening the eyes. Every 500 grams of shepherd's purse contains 25.2 grams of protein and 12.8 grams of carotene, ranking them as the best vegetable sources of these ingredients. Shepherd's purse is also higher in vitamin C than many citrus fruits. It is also high in riboflavin, also known as vitamin B2. Shepherd's purse also has one of the highest protein contents of any non-leguminous vegetable. It also contains fat, calcium, phosphorus, iron and a large amount of fiber and vitamins. The climate is dry in spring, so it is very important to recuperate the liver and lungs. Shepherd's purse is a great food for softening the liver and nourishing the lungs in spring, and can be put into soups and stir-fries or as a filling for ravioli or pies. After washing, scald it with boiling water, squeeze the water and store it in the refrigerator, and take it whenever you need. In the spring when the climate is highly changeable, eating shepherd's purse can effectively prevent and treat many common diseases, such as influenza, epidemic meningitis and conjunctivitis. It is also useful in the prevention and treatment of osteomalacia, measles, skin keratosis, respiratory infections, prostatitis, urinary infections and so on. According to TCM ideology, the shepherd's purse is a combination of sweet, tasteless flavors, and slightly cold properties. This means it helps cool the blood for hemostasis, promotes urination and eliminates dampness, and removes liver fire for improving eyesight. It can be used to treat female metrorrhagia, menorrhagia, hematuria, hemoptysis, heat strangury, edema, difficulties urinating, cloudy urine, leucorrhea and other diseases. Shepherd's purse is thus sometimes referred to as a good medicine for gynecology. It is particularly useful for the elderly.

Leeks: Traditional Chinese medicine believes that leeks have warming effects on the kidneys, spleen and stomach, promoting *qi* and blood circulation. This helps reduce levels of fat in the blood and promote the healthy operation of the stomach and intestines. Leeks are a great food for the kidneys. Eating leeks in spring will help strengthen the kidneys, however those with hyperactive fire elements in their body due to *yin* deficiencies (symptoms include irritability, flushing on cheeks, hypersexuality) should be careful of how much they eat. In addition, leeks should not be eaten with hard liquor, since hard liquors are hot in nature while leeks are warm and pungent. Eating both together is like adding fuel to a fire.

Celery: In spring, which is typically a vegetable off-season, fresh green celery is especially popular. This is not only because it is fragrant and delicious. It can be stir-fried, eaten cold, and also used as a filling. There are many ways to consume celery, and it has high nutritional and therapeutic value. Celery contains a variety of nutrients that are beneficial to the human body, including very high levels of protein and twice the amount of phosphorus found in cucurbits. Celery also has high levels of calcium and iron, 20 times more than tomatoes. Celery leaf is also very nutritionally rich. According to analysis, for 10 out of 13 nutritional components found in celery, there are significantly higher levels found in the leaf than in the stem. Celery also has an attractive aromatic smell, which can stimulate and increase the appetite as well as strengthen the spleen. Eating celery regularly can promote children's growth and development, and can also alleviate many health issues common amongst the middle-aged and elderly, such as arteriosclerosis, neurasthenia, constipation and so on. According to TCM, liver *yang* is easily hyperactive and liver wind can easily strike in spring, which can cause flare-ups in patients with high blood pressure and even cause stroke if their mood fluctuates severely. Celery is sweet and cool in properties and has the effect of calming liver *yang* and lowering blood pressure. For the treatment of high blood pressure, wash and boil 250 grams of fresh celery before chopping and mashing it to squeeze out the juice. Drink one small cup twice a day. Generally, this treatment should be used for seven days. After four weeks of continuous use, it can be drunk once a day. Long-term consumption can help keep blood pressure stable.

Honey

In spring, many people suffer from excessive thirst, coughs, constipation and other ailments. Individuals with weaker constitutions may also find they are frequently infected with viruses, and are vulnerable to hepatitis, tuberculosis and other infectious diseases. One underrated way to prevent these diseases is to eat more nourishing and detoxifying foods in spring. Honey is one of these foods.

Chinese Wolfberry

In the early spring, Chinese wolfberry (also known as lycium barbarum) sprouts tender seedlings, which are slightly bitter but very refreshing. These seedlings can clear bodily fire elements and brighten the eyes. This plant is commonly used in folklore to treat *yin* deficiency and internal heat, dry and painful throat, excessive liver fire, dizziness, low fevers and so on. Wolfberry is rich in nutrients, containing 4 g of protein, 0.8 g of fat, 19.3 g of sugar, 55 mg of calcium, 86 mg of phosphorus, 8.6 mg of carotene and various vitamins per 100 grams. Twenty grams of it brewed in hot water to make a tea is beneficial to patients with high blood pressure and diabetes. The wolfberry fruit and black plum ground together and brewed with boiling water into a mixture can relieve summer-heat and thirst.

Pineapple

Pineapple is rich in fructose, glucose, amino acids, organic acids, vitamins and other nutrients. The calcium content is twice that of bananas, and five times that of grapes, the phosphorus content is three times that of apples and five times that of pears, and the vitamin C content is far more than that of summer fruits such as peaches, plums and apricots. Pineapple's vitamin B1 content is second only to citrus.

Pineapple is generally eaten raw, but can also be cooked with other fruits to make a soup, or cooked with fish. According to TCM, the color and flavor elements of pineapple enter into the Taiyin Spleen Meridian of Foot (SP), which has the effects of nourishing the spleen and replenishing *qi*. It also helps your appetite and digestion, as it helps produce saliva and slake the thirst. Eating pineapple can also relieve greasiness and aid digestion. Pineapple also contains an enzyme that can dissolve blood clots, helping those that consume it avoid blood vessel obstruction, protecting the heart and preventing heart disease.

Here are a few easy ways to incorporate highly nutritious pineapple into your diet and help prevent digestive tract diseases: Take one pineapple and two oranges. Peel, chop and juice them. Mix the two juices together, and drink 20 ml of the resulting juice twice a day to combat indigestion. Alternatively, take one pineapple and cut it into small pieces to eat three times a day; this can help treat dysentery. Another option is to eat 30 grams of boiled pineapple leaves, twice a day. This can help treat enteritis that causes diarrhea.

Pineapple must be soaked in salt water first, to remove proteases and glycosides. This helps avoid allergic reactions and any discomfort in the mouth.

Herbal Teas for Spring

Spring is the season of recovery, when ice thaws and snow melts. The human body, just like nature, is also in a phase of relaxation. However, at this time, people often report feeling sleepy and weak. In addition, the weather is very changeable at this time, which brings opportunities for germs to invade the human body. It is therefore a good time to brew plenty of healthy herbal teas at home and drink them regularly. This works to not only eliminate springtime lethargy, but also helps strengthen the body's natural resistance to infection and disease, improving your overall health, longevity, skin and other health indicators.

① Dandelion Tea

Ingredients: 20 g dandelion, 15 g honey, 3 g licorice, 15–20 g green tea

Method: First, brew the dandelion, licorice and green tea in water for 15 minutes, and then add honey to the decoction before drinking.

Effects: Clears heat and removes toxicity. Used to treat colds caused by wind heat, fever, non-severe aversion to wind cold, problem sweating, headaches, nasal congestion, dry mouth, slight thirst, sore and swollen throat and other ailments.

② Three-Flower Tea

Ingredients: 15 g honeysuckle, 10 g chrysanthemum, 3 g jasmine

Method: Put the three flowers into the teacup, soak them in boiling water, and serve as tea.

Effects: Clears heat and removes toxicity. Used to treat colds caused by wind heat, fever, non-severe aversion to wind cold, sweating, nasal congestion, sore and swollen throat and other ailments.

③ Monk Fruit Tea

Ingredients: 20 g siraitia grosvenorii (monk fruit, or *luo han guo* in Chinese), 2 g green tea

Method: First add 300–500 ml water to the monk fruit, boil for five to ten minutes, add the green tea, and then cover and simmer for one to two minutes.

Effects: Clears heat, reduces phlegm, and relieves coughs. Used to treat colds caused by wind-heat, yellow phlegm or whooping cough in children.

④ Fat Burning Tea

Ingredients: 30 g fresh hawthorn berries, 6 g Sophora japonica flowers, 10 g poria cocos, rock sugar

Method: Pit and mash the hawthorn berries, and then put them into a pot with the poria cocos. Add some water, simmer for about ten minutes, and remove any bits, leaving the pure juice. Soak the Sophora japonica flowers with this juice, and sweeten it with sugar to taste.

Effects: Improves appetite and helps digestion. Also helps reduce blood pressure and cholesterol, relaxing the blood vessels and guarding against stroke.

⑤ Rose Tea

Ingredients: 3–5 g dried roses

Method: Brew the dried roses in hot water to make a simple tea.

Effects: Helps cool the blood, nourish the skin, aid digestion and burn fat, aiding weight loss. Best drunk after meals. Rose tea has a strong floral fragrance, meaning it also helps combat bad breath.

⑥ Dried Orange Peel and Ginger Tea

Ingredients: 20 g dried orange peel, 10 g fresh sliced ginger,

5 g licorice root, 5 g tea leaf

Method: Bring a pot of water to a boil, then put the dried orange peel, ginger slices, licorice root and tea into it. Brew for about ten minutes, and then remove any residue, leaving the liquid.

Effects: Relieves coughs, strengthens the stomach and aids digestion.

Medicinal Food Recipes

① Chrysanthemum and Coix Seed Soup

Ingredients: 50 g coix seeds, three to five dried chrysanthemum flowers

Method: Soak the coix seeds for at least one hour, and then heat the water to boil until the coix seeds are soft. Add three to five dried chrysanthemums flowers, and simmer together for another five minutes.

Effects: Many elderly people have a persistent bitter taste in the mouth though they haven't eaten anything bitter. *Su Wen*, one of China's most famous ancient medicinal texts and a part of *The Yellow Emperor's Classic of Medicine*, states that "liver heat is expressed via excessive bile, resulting in bitterness in the mouth." So, to get rid of the bitter taste, it is necessary to deal with the liver and gall heat. Drinking chrysanthemum and coix seed soup is a good method for this. Chrysanthemum has slightly cold properties, which help relieve liver fire and clear gallbladder heat; coix seed is of cool properties, and helps invigorate the spleen and clear heat from the body.

② Ginger and Glutinous Rice Porridge

Ingredients: 3–5 g fresh ginger, 50–100 g glutinous rice, five to six stems of spring onion with roots, 10–15 ml rice vinegar

Method: Wash the glutinous rice and ginger and put them into a pot. Bring to the boil once or twice, then add the spring onion stems. Once the porridge is ready, add the rice vinegar, and simmer to taste.

Effects: Relieves superficies syndrome and dispels coldness.

The effects are the most ideal for colds caused by wind cold and flu in spring. The soup should be drunk while hot. Lie down and rest after consumption for the best effects.

③ Quail Egg Soup

Ingredients: 10 g angelica sinensis, 10 g astragalus root, ten quail eggs

Method: Cook all ingredients in boiling water.

Effects: Replenishes the blood and *qi*, and strengthens the body. Helps prevent a variety of infectious diseases.

④ Spring Onion, Ginger and Coriander Soup

Ingredients: 15–30 g stems of spring onion with roots, 10–20 g ginger, 10–15 g coriander, 10–30 ml rice vinegar

Method: First, decoct the ginger in water for about five minutes, then add spring onion stems and coriander, and decoct for a further two to four minutes. Then, add the rice vinegar, remove all ingredients, and consume the soup while hot. This is a fresh-tasting soup and should not be cooked for long.

Effects: Relieves superficies syndrome and dispels coldness. Highly effective in treating wind-cold illnesses in their early stages. After consumption, lie down under bed covers to aid sweating.

⑤ Chinese Wolfberry and White Fungus Soup

Ingredients: 10 g Chinese white fungus, 10 g wolfberry, 15 g yam, 3 g chrysanthemum, 30 g rock sugar, two egg whites

Method: Stew the white fungus, wolfberry and yam with water. Add the rock sugar and egg whites, then sprinkle with chrysanthemum, and simmer slightly.

Effects: Nourishes the spleen, strengthens the stomach and strengthens vital *qi*. Also helps prevent infectious diseases such as meningitis and scarlet fever.

⑥ Water Chestnut and Radish Juice

Ingredients: 250 g water chestnut, 250 g radish

Method: Wash ingredients. Squeeze the juice from them separately, then mix well and drink as desired.

Effects: Strengthens the spleen and stomach. Helps prevent

whooping cough, diphtheria and other diseases.

⑦ Bacon and Onion Soup

Ingredients: two bacon slices, one onion, one teaspoon soy sauce, 1.5 bowls of water, a little salt

Method: Cut the bacon into thin strips. Remove the outer layers of the onion and cut it into thin shreds. Heat the bacon in a deep pan on low heat until fragrant, then add the onion and stir continuously. Add the soy sauce and salt and continue to stir on low heat until the onion is soft. Add the bowl and a half of water, then simmer on low heat for about 15 minutes.

Effects: Antibacterial. Also helps improve immune response, preventing infectious diseases in spring.

⑧ Cool Yam and Wolfberry Mix

Ingredients: 200 g yam, 6 g wolfberry

Method: Remove the peel of yam. Mix together sliced yam and wolfberry, or add some coconut milk.

Effects: Strengthens the stomach and intestines, improves immune response and helps prevent infectious diseases in spring.

⑨ Dandelion and Chinese Ballon Flower Soup

Ingredients: 60 g dandelion, 10 g Chinese balloon flower (Platycodon grandiflorus), a little white sugar

Method: Mix the above ingredients together and boil them into a soup.

Effects: Reduces swelling and oozing. Also helps combat carbuncles.

⑩ Dandelion and Corn Soup

Ingredients: 60 g dandelion, 60 g corn cob

Method: Drink the decoction of the above ingredients, or drink it instead of tea.

Effects: Acts as a diuretic, freeing strangury. Used to treat heat strangury and brown-colored urine of reduced amount.

5. Spring Lifestyle

During the spring, taking care of your sleep pattern and lifestyle is just as important as diet for protecting your health. Making sure you sleep six to eight hours a night is crucial, and you should also aim to get plenty of time outside in natural light, breathing fresh air.

Recommended Sleeping Patterns

Chinese medicine believes that in spring, the best sleeping pattern is to sleep slightly later and rise early. Once winter has passed, the days are longer and nights shorter. According to the theory outlined in *The Yellow Emperor's Classic of Medicine*, humans should fall in with this natural rhythm change, moderately reducing our sleeping times and increasing our activity.

The generation and reduction of *yang qi* in our body are closely related to sleep. When we are awake, *yang qi* expresses and moves externally. When we fall asleep, it moves inside the body. Therefore, if we want the body's *yang qi* to reflect that of nature, we must reduce our sleeping hours to reflect the reduced hours of the night. Too much sleep can easily cause the body's *yang qi* to stagnate, which is not conducive to the age-old concept in Chinese medicine of "nourishing *yang* in spring and summer."

Although you should go to bed later and get up earlier in spring, don't overdo it; wake early, but not before five o'clock. Bedtimes should not be later than 11 o'clock. Too little sleep is very harmful to human health.

Dressing Comfortably

In spring, you should make an effort to loosen your hair, loosen buttons, stretch your body frequently and walk around your home. This helps quickly activate your mind. It's also important for clothes not to be too tight in spring. Younger people, especially young women, may be tempted to switch thicker winter pants for tighter pants or leggings in spring before the weather has sufficiently warmed, but this should be avoided if your goal is optimal health. One crucial but often overlooked reason for this is that the female crotch area should not be clothed too tightly. Tight-fitting pants or leggings can stop the vagina from properly secreting acidic fluids that help keep it clean and bacteria-free. Moreover, they're unhelpful in keeping the vulva dry. Additionally, if the vulva is exposed to excessive heat and humidity for long periods of time, this creates favorable conditions for bacterial reproduction and can easily cause inflammation. Loose, comfortable clothing is recommended.

Keeping Warm
Traditional Chinese health ideology emphasizes wrapping up against cold in spring. This is because, although winter has finished, people's metabolic function and disease resistance is still in their winter phase. The purpose of staying wrapped up is to protect people from colds, which they are especially vulnerable to in this period because heat production in the body has decreased. It can be tempting to shed your layers as soon as spring begins to warm the air, but this should be done with caution. Too much cold air exposure increases blood flow resistance, affecting the body's functions and potentially opening the door to disease. For this reason, you should always try to keep warm in spring, especially early in the morning and late at night. It is a good idea to wear extra layers and sleep with enough blankets, making sure your back and legs are covered to preserve your *yang qi* and enhance immunity.

Looking After Your Nose
The weather is changeable in early spring, with temperatures often varying more than 10℃ one day to the next. During this time, the *yin* cold of winter has not yet completely given way to the *yang qi*. The human body's resistance to wind pathogens is weakened, making it easy to get sick. The nose is an open window into the respiratory system, and is connected to the ears and throat, which means nose infection can also cause ear and throat diseases, and even affect the upper respiratory tract.

This is why traditional Chinese medicine believes it is crucial to properly "protect the nose in spring."

One specific method for this is to hold warm water or warm salt water in the palm, lower the head and inhale it through the nose. Afterwards, you should spit out the residue of this through the mouth or blow it out through the nose. This can be repeated several times. You might also use a bottle of warm saline solution and a tube inserted 2–3 cm into your nasal cavity, rinsing and blowing your nose to wash it out. Consistently performing this cleaning routine has significant protective effects.

Fresh Air
Open doors and windows and let more sunlight and air into the house, helping keep indoor air fresh and clean. Frequently cleaning and making sure dirt is removed even from room corners helps minimize bacteria and reduce airborne pollution. In China's "plum rain" season, dampness and mildew are common. Wherever you are in the world, there is likely to be a season of heavier rain; this advice is applicable to that season for you. This refers to June to July in southern China, and the period is so named because plums indigenous to this region ripen. During this period of frequent rain, it is advisable to use vinegar and mugwort to disinfect and dehumidify houses. Method: Use 5–10 ml vinegar for each cubic meter of space. Add 10–20 ml water to dilute the vinegar, heat the mixture, then put it in a container and allow it to evaporate in a room for two hours. This should be done once every other day, three to five times in total. You can also burn dried mugwort or moxa sticks one to two times a day, for about 20 minutes each time.

The occurrence of colds is related to poor air circulation. The main way that cold viruses spread is via droplets. This means that any situation in which indoor air does not circulate properly, or where many people live close together, is a high-risk environment for cross-infection. Therefore, the prevention of colds rests not only on preventive medicines, but also on the environment. Make sure you keep fresh air circulating, and breathe as much fresh air as possible. You can also spend less time in communal places.

Foot Soaks

In early spring, it's important to keep your feet warm as the temperature fluctuates between cold and hot. Because the feet are an extremity, they are part of the body that is furthest from the heart. This means they have less blood supply. Additionally, they have very little fat around them, making them vulnerable to the cold. If the feet get cold, they are particularly prone to causing constriction of capillary vessels in the upper respiratory tract, leading to a decline in immunity. The respiratory tract is extremely sensitive to cold air. A sudden drop in temperature can reduce the resistance of the respiratory organs, and pathogens can take advantage of this. It can cause coughs in mild cases and respiratory diseases such as bronchitis and asthma in severe cases.

Therefore, if conditions permit, it is best to soak your feet in hot water before traveling. Soaking feet in hot water can not only prevent respiratory diseases, but also make blood vessels dilate, improving blood flow. This improves skin condition and tissue nutrition, reducing the occurrence of lower limb aches and giving people more energy. Adding in a few herbal ingredients to the water can also help treat tinea pedis.

Leek herbal foot soak: Boil a small handful of leeks in one liter of water and simmer for six minutes. Soak feet for more than half an hour every day for a week for one course of treatment.

Sichuan pepper herbal foot soak: Take about ten whole Sichuan peppers, place them into a basin, and use boiling water to brew. Leave water until it cools to a warm temperature. When it is less than 40℃ , you can soak your feet. Use once a week for several weeks. This has a good effect on relieving tinea pedis and treating sweaty feet.

6. Emotional Health in Spring

People's mental and emotional well-being is collectively referred to as their emotional health in traditional Chinese medicine. Chinese medicine believes that there are seven emotions and six desires that every person has. Emotions are normal physiological phenomena, which act as protective reactions to external and internal stimuli. They are beneficial to physical and mental health. However, emotional instability and excessive emotions can lead to physical and mental disorders. The ability to regulate your emotions is, therefore, of great benefit to your health. Nourishing your mind and calming your spirit will allow you to maintain a happy and contented mood at all times. The liver controls conveyance and dispersion of *qi* and emotion. In spring, the liver *yang* moves easily, making many people more irritable. Therefore, we can see that the regulation of our emotions helps prevent disease caused by abnormal *qi* movements in the body or hepatic disorder. In order to do this, in spring, you should aim to keep your mood stable and relaxed, ensuring that your liver can function properly, eliminating disease and strengthening your body.

A Peaceful State of Mind

First of all, regulation of one's emotions helps avoid damage to the liver. For people prone to either depression or irritability, this is a crucial component of spring health care. For these two groups of people, there are traditional Chinese medicines that can be used to help soothe the liver, regulating *qi* and clearing heat.

In spring, those who feel depressed should fill their diet with fragrant and fresh fennel, radish and orange. Take and brew ten grams of astragalus, three slices of ginger, and five jujubes, and the decoction can be drunk as tea. Those who feel easily irritable should eat bitter and sour foods such as balsam pear and hawthorn berries. They should also take and brew ten grams of chrysanthemum, ten grams of cassia seeds and three grams of licorice root and drink the decoction as tea.

Reducing Stress

Traditional Chinese medicine always emphasizes the ideology of
"treating the mind first, and then the body." With the increasing
competition in modern life, chronic stress and depression are
real health issues for great numbers of people. It is common for
patients to experience flare-ups of old diseases due to current
emotional states. Many patients know intuitively that their
illness is related to their emotions, but do not know how to
"reduce" their negative emotions. People of different age groups
tend to face different types of stress and pressure. We give the
following advice to different groups:

Those who are middle-aged often have both dependent
children and elderly, as well as professional struggles. The pressure
is enormous, and this group is often understandably exhausted.
People's energy reserves are not infinite. If you are middle-
aged, you must learn to understand the balance and relationship
between your energy levels and stress levels. Overthinking is
a quick way to damage your state of mind. It's important to
prioritize a balance between mental and physical strength. When
the brain is used excessively, stress can be relieved by increasing
physical exercise and making sure you're sleeping enough. Good
sleep is a highly effective way to relieve psychological stress.
Generally, you should sleep from 10 pm to 6 am.

For the elderly, the most important thing is to be contented
and happy, and maintain a positive mindset. According to *The
Yellow Emperor's Classic of Medicine*, too much desire can cause
anxiety, irritability, and emotional uneasiness, which will lead to
deficiencies of nutrient-blood, sluggish defensive *qi* and related
diseases.

In short, your mindset being off can quickly result in reduced
immunity, cardio-cerebrovascular diseases, stomach problems
and mental disorders. So when caring for our health in spring,
mood regulation is key. You should make an effort to control
your anger and reduce irritability, keeping yourself calm,
open-minded and optimistic, and above all stable.

Learning to Accept Imperfection

When working on one's mental health, it is important to self-reflect, and not to blame others. You must learn to be tolerant of things not going your way, so that you can remain detached and polite. Do not spend time arguing over trivial things, and let go of your need to be competitive. Take time to recognize your strengths and weaknesses, and treat both your work and private life with a calm attitude.

7. Physiotherapy and Health in Spring

In the spring, people are often early on in their work year, and are working hard. Professional stress can easily build up. This time of year, the days are longer and nights shorter, and temperatures can vary largely. Many people report more sickness at this time of year, with complaints such as tension headaches, arthritis, colds, etc. Traditional Chinese medicine recommends the use of moxibustion, massage and other physical therapies to drive away these complaints. Massage can play a highly effective therapeutic role by regulating the nervous system. Massage is very relaxing and non-invasive.

Moxibustion

Yang qi ascends in spring, making it a good time to cultivate positive *yang* energy. However, many people make the mistake of not keeping warm enough through the winter, resulting in them losing much of their *yang qi*. In spring, we can make up this loss by using moxibustion to help eliminate deficient and cold pathogens in the body. Moxibustion (mugwort burning) can warm and replenish *qi* and blood, and can also regulate *qi* movement, encouraging the body's natural health regulation.

Method: Burn a moxa stick over the Shenque acupoint (the navel). Fumigating the Shenque acupoint with moxa sticks in early spring helps mobilize *yang qi* in the body, which is very good for health. Please note that this method should be avoided during menstruation and pregnancy.

Although moxibustion has very good health benefits, you must be careful to do it at the right time when treating some diseases and syndromes. For insomnia, moxibustion should be done before going to bed. Do not utilize moxibustion before meals or immediately after meals, and do not do it for long to begin with.

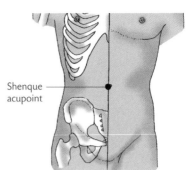

Shenque acupoint

Massaging

Spring is a high-incidence season for the flu, so it is very important to do a good job at prevention. Massaging

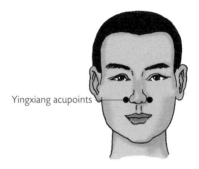

Yingxiang acupoints

the Yingxiang acupoints is effective in the elimination and prevention of cold symptoms.

Location of the Yingxiang acupoints: On the face, in the creases about 1 cm away from the edge of your nose (in the nasolabial groove).

Massage method: Press the Yingxiang acupoints on both sides of the nose with the index finger of both hands, and rub them in clockwise and counterclockwise directions 36 times respectively. You should feel a slight soreness that radiates up to your forehead and cheeks.

Frequent massage of Yingxiang acupoints can enhance your resistance to pathogens, and also promote blood circulation around the nose, unblocking *qi* and blood flow. This helps your body protect itself.

Chapter Two
Summer

Summer is a season of prosperity and beauty. The heaven's *qi* falls, the earth's *qi* rises, and the energy of heaven and earth mingles, while plants bloom and bear fruit. At this time, the earth is lush and the sun is bright. Nature is full of vitality, and growth comes easily. Life is at its peak. Heat and humidity are the main characteristics of summer. The weather gets hotter by the week. If you live in an area with a summer rainy season, then the humidity is also likely to be very high. In these common cases, the following principles should be followed to make sure you are maximizing your health outcomes.

Nourishing *yin* and reinforcing *yang*: This is determined by the climate characteristics of summer. Summer-heat pathogens, sometimes called "heatstroke" in English, and dampness pathogens are both "pathogenic *qi*," although their natures are opposite to one another. Summer-heat is a "*yang* pathogen," and can easily damage and consume the body's clear fluid and resulting in "heat change" in the body. Popular methods to cope with this are to avoid the heat, nourish *yin* and generate clear fluid. Dampness is a "*yin* pathogen" characterized by downward movement, heavy textures and a turbid nature. According to traditional Chinese medicine, dampness is an "earth" energy. Since the spleen is an earth organ, damp *qi* is on the same scale, so dampness can easily get trapped in the spleen and cause *qi* blockages. When energy is trapped in the spleen in this way, it can cause pain in the intestines and stomach. You may have no appetite with abdominal distension, loose stool, or get cold limbs. Clearly, then, *yang* reinforcement is vital in this season.

Strengthening the spleen and stomach: In summer,

people tend to drink more water, and the spleen and stomach are often working overtime to process this water and hydrate the body. The spleen and stomach, therefore, need to be in good condition. Looking after them properly is crucial. To do this, it's a good idea to eat some pungent seasonings, such as pepper, coriander, garlic, vinegar, ginger, scallions, and so on. Balsam pear is also a good ingredient to use. When it's hot outside, people tend to crave cold drinks, but consuming anything ice cold should be done with caution. Drinking too much of anything ice cold can hurt the stomach and spleen. Anything iced should be consumed slowly and steadily, not gulped down or eaten too fast. Massaging the abdomen (do not massage when full or hungry) and the Zusanli acupoints can also help strengthen the spleen and stomach.

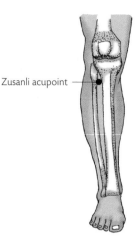

Zusanli acupoint

Clearing and nourishing the heart: The season of summer corresponds to the "fire" element, and the "heart" organ. However, summer is also the season in which the heart must work hardest. Hot weather accelerates the blood flow in the body, so the workload of the heart is increased. It's also very easy to get over-excited in the summer-heat, a condition known in Chinese medicine as excessive heart fire. This heart fire should be controlled. To do this, we should first learn to avoid the heat. Avoid very crowded places. Second, ensure adequate sleep. One can sleep late before 23:00, and take a nap between 11:00 and 13:00. Utilize cool-natured foods, such as lotus seed porridge, lily porridge, mung bean soup, and red bean soup. You should also be aware of the raised risk for epidemic encephalitis B, heatstroke, diarrhea and other summer diseases. The first aspect of health in summer is the focus on keeping your diet clean, not spending too long in the sun, and creating a comfortable microclimate for yourself. The second is ensuring that the spleen, stomach, heart and lungs function properly and can resist pathogenic *qi*. Covering both of these bases is a good approach to summertime health.

1. Prevention in Summer

In summer, health preservation is based on regulating the spirit, maintaining a happy and stable mood, and avoiding large emotional ups and downs, as these add internal heat to an already hot season. Good health preservation can be achieved by calming the mind. This is supplemented by paying attention to nutrition. Diet is very effective in the prevention and treatment of common summertime ailments.

Summer is the season with the highest temperature of the year, and the metabolism of the human body works in overdrive. In the heat, many people experience fatigue, loss of appetite, sweating, dizziness, anxiety and drowsiness, or may even suffer from more serious ailments such as heatstroke, vomiting, abdominal pain and diarrhea. So what does it take to stay healthy in summer?

Heatstroke

In summer, both dry heat and humid heat can cause heatstroke, especially for people working outdoors. Heatstroke is an acute disease occurring in summer or high-temperature environments. The first signs are fever, dizziness, thirst, fatigue, and lack of sweat. This is followed by high fever, dizziness, irritability, convulsions and cold limbs. If untreated, heatstroke can be fatal. Heatstroke has an acute onset, can change rapidly, and has a powerful impact on the body's clear fluid and *qi*. The disease is mainly linked to high-temperature environments and the difficulty of sweat evaporating from the body. This leads to a large increase in the body's heat production, and this heat builds and builds until it is at dangerous levels.

If signs of heatstroke appear, sufferers should be moved to a cool place, and their collar loosened to ensure smooth breathing. If possible, compress a towel soaked in hot water on the navel, and administer ten drops of water (TCM herb *shi di shui*) or Huoxiang Zhengqi Powder orally. Alternatively, use a *gua sha* board or a gauze sterilized with alcohol to scrape both sides of the back, ribs or forehead in a vertical motion until the skin goes a dark purple color. You might also apply cooling oil before scraping.

People with less robust physiques should avoid walking in the hot sun for too long and use plenty of sunscreens. Applying cooling oil on your forehead can also prevent heatstroke. The following measures can also be taken to prevent heatstroke in summer:

① Wear sunglasses, caps or use a parasol when going out.

② Clothes should be light in color and made of translucent cotton or silk fabrics. Anyone out on a bike for a long time in the hot sun should wear long-sleeved clothing.

③ Patients with hypertension, coronary heart disease, cerebral arteriosclerosis and other diseases should not stay in air-conditioned rooms for too long to prevent flare-ups of old diseases. Pay attention to ventilation in air-conditioned rooms. The temperature should not be set too low.

④ Anyone planning on being outdoors for a long time should take heatstroke prevention medicine with them.

⑤ Make sure you eat adequate protein. Your daily protein intake should be increased by 10% to 15% in summer. Fresh fish, shrimp, chicken, duck and other high-quality protein foods with low-fat content are all good choices. You might also eat more soybean products or other foods rich in plant protein.

⑥ In case of excessive sweating, make sure you supplement your sodium and potassium. Sodium can be supplemented by eating a little more salt or soy sauce with your food. Foods with high potassium content include bananas, bean products, kelp, etc.

⑦ Drink water constantly. Don't wait until you are thirsty.

⑧ Don't overdo it with cold drinks. Too much of them can restrict blood flow in your gut and affect digestive function.

⑨ It's a good idea to eat more fleshy vegetables such as cucumbers and squashes. Eat more foods of a cool nature, including vegetables such as tomato, eggplant, lettuce and asparagus. Bitter foods should also be consumed. This includes sowthistle, bitter bamboo shoots, etc.

⑩ Do not drink spirits.

⑪ Bathe regularly, always wiping your skin with a wet towel.

⑫ Make sure you're sleeping enough and resting when you feel tired.

Problems Caused by Air Conditioning

"Air-conditioning syndrome" is a general term for a set of symptoms, rather than a medically defined disease. In summer, high temperatures can be unbearable, and the modern air conditioner (AC) has become one of the most frequently used household appliances. In order to keep cool, many people keep their AC on at home all night, only to find when they get up the next morning that they have a sore throat. As well as this, excessive use of AC can cause colds, facial paralysis, skin allergies, pneumonia and other diseases or related symptoms. This has a significant effect on health, which is why the symptoms are sometimes known as air-conditioning syndrome.

When staying in air-conditioned rooms, you should drink more water, and take in more vitamins. Air conditioners should also have their temperature kept at about 26℃ to prevent excessive indoor and outdoor temperature differences. Individuals should make sure they spend no more time in air-conditioned rooms than is necessary for work and sleep. It's also a good idea to engage in more outdoor activities. Those who have chronic cough symptoms or who are allergic to cold air should be well aware of their physical conditions and use air conditioning as little as they can.

It is easy to impair the flow of *qi* in the summer, which can limit physical strength and vitality. This is manifested as excessive sweating. If your body does not replace lost water in a timely manner, this can damage clear fluid production. For patients with cardio-cerebrovascular issues, summertime is a risky period for cardiac function because of this possible disruption of clear fluid and *qi*. Therefore, we should pay special attention to "nourishing *qi*" in summer to prevent the lack of *yang qi* in the coming winter. To nourish *qi*, we must mind the difference between body temperature and room temperature. Air conditioning should be set to around 26℃, ensuring the temperature is not too low. We must make sure that we spend the summer in a moderately cool, dry and comfortable environment, and avoid all kinds of diseases caused by coolness.

Diarrhea

Diarrhea is one of the most common complaints of summer. In the summer heat, many people crave ice-cold drinks, but drinking them at a time of year when the gastrointestinal function is fragile, or while maintaining an unhygienic diet, can cause acute stomach problems. Bacterial stomach infections, indigestion and other stomach issues are all common, and can lead to diarrhea. In summer, gastrointestinal discomfort, diarrhea and vomiting can be caused by rapid changes in weather, excessive use of air conditioning, eating iced fruit, carsickness and seasickness, and acclimatization. Traditional Chinese medicine attributes these ailments to internal damage and excessive dampness, and can be categorized as a type of non-bacterial gastrointestinal diseases. Taking antibiotics to deal with this kind of complaint is therefore not only ineffective, but can damage your gut biome, aggravating the problem. Huoxiang Zhengqi Powder helps regulate dampness, harmonizing the stomach and strengthening the spleen. It can have a significant effect against non-bacterial gastrointestinal diseases, and is a good first choice for regulating gastrointestinal discomfort in summer.

Many children also have diarrhea problems in summer, because children's gastrointestinal tract is more sensitive. Diarrhea is often accompanied by vomiting, and it can be hard for children to keep the medicine down. Be aware that imprudent use of antibiotics is likely to cause antibiotic resistance, worsening the problem in the long term. Traditional Chinese medicine asserts that diarrhea in babies in summer is also mainly caused by overeating and damp-heat. If the baby's stool has a sour smell, and is mixed with food residue, accompanied by nausea and vomiting, this can be attributed to food-related diarrhea. If the baby's stool is yellow, thin, frequent, the anus is red, and the tongue coating is yellow, this means it is damp-heat diarrhea.

Infants with diarrhea should be given some lightly salted water. If the baby has a lot of diarrhea, accompanied by frequent vomiting, thirst, irritability, a lack of spirit and other dehydration symptoms, he should see a doctor immediately and undergo rehydration treatment.

Excessive Internal Heat

In summer, many people suffer from a dry mouth, mouth ulcers, dark yellow urine, dry stools and other internal heat-related symptoms. To combat this, it is necessary to master some heatstroke prevention skills, to help remove some heart fire and recuperate the body and mind.

A calm mind relieves summer-heat. When it comes to looking after one's spirit, the ancient Chinese treatise on health preservation, the *Yang Sheng Lun* or *Discussions on Health Preservation* emphasizes that "it is best to regulate and calm the mind in summer, like placing ice and snow in the heart, to reduce heat in one's heart." It is particularly important in this season to be calm at all times, which is the reason why so many of China's ancients advocated a "calm and collected" approach to life.

Bitter foods soothe heart fire. A preventative diet is always better than medicine, and this logic holds true in summer. Traditional Chinese medicine believes that the four seasons and five flavors correspond to the viscera of the human body. In summer, a small amount of bitter food adds a little of the "bitter" element to the heart organ, and can reduce heart fire. Bitter foods include vegetables such as balsam pear, lettuce, fennel, radish leaves, sowthistle, etc. Fruits include apricot, grapefruit, citrus, aloe, etc. Drinks include Kuding tea, tartary buckwheat tea, etc. However, bitter food is not suitable for everyone. Traditional Chinese medicine believes that bitter and cold foods can be hard on the stomach, and people with spleen and stomach deficiency should not eat too much of them. This can easily cause nausea, vomiting, diarrhea and other adverse consequences. In addition, bitter products can easily produce dryness and damage the body's *yin* and fluid. People with *yin* deficiencies should therefore eat less bitter food.

Massage can help soothe the mind and spirit. Massaging acupoints can also clear heart fire and calm the spirit. For example, acupoints such as the Shenting, Baihui and Taiyang on the head, Hegu on the hands, and Taichong on the insteps all help regulate the circulation of *qi* and blood in the liver meridian. They can also help lower *qi* in the heart. Similarly, a "patting" massage performed on the armpits can also relieve heat in the body. The Jiquan acupoints in the armpits are located at the place where you can feel a pulse, at the top of the armpits. Massage method: Raise the left hand, palm up, and pat the left armpit with the right palm. Then, lift your right hand up and slap your right armpit with the palm of your left hand, 30 to 50 times per set. Perform five sets.

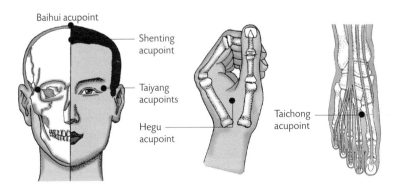

Baihui acupoint
Shenting acupoint
Taiyang acupoints
Hegu acupoint
Taichong acupoint

Pompholyx

Hot and humid weather is likely to cause some eczema and atopic dermatitis. Amongst these, pompholyx is the most common. In summer, not only the body is prone to sweat, but also the hands are prone to sweat. Many people's palms are wet at most times. In addition to an unpleasant look, blisters also itch. In severe cases, sufferers may encounter secondary infection, which leads to swelling and pain in the hands. Chinese ancients believed that groups of small blisters on the palms of hands and feet were caused by hyperhidrosis and a poorly regulated sweating system. It usually occurs on the side of the palm or between the fingers. When you squeeze these blisters, you will find that the liquid inside is clear, or occasionally not clear. When it dries up, it will peel off and reveal new, pink skin, but this skin cracks easily and can be painful. These blisters usually appear in the late spring and early summer. In summer, the disease worsens and attacks repeatedly. It can last for a long time.

In summer, people often eat inappropriately. Many eat too much cold food, or eat too much fatty, sweet or rich food, such as greasy fried and barbecued food. These types of foods cause the internal retention of damp-heat, which damages the spleen and stomach. In addition, if the weather is hot and an individual's state of mind is depressed, irritable or anxious, this will further strain the heart and spleen. In this scenario, the spleen can begin to function abnormally. Heat and dampness gather together in the body. When combined with the extra effect of heat and humidity outside, the skin cannot get rid of the heat. It flows to the palms along the meridians, and causes sweat blisters. What can we do to remove dampness, clear heat and stop itching? Now is a good time to introduce some acupoints.

Massage of the Laogong acupoint: Press on the Laogong acupoint, found in the palm of the right hand, with the tip of the left thumb. Press it vertically downward, and press the rest of the fingers on the back of the hand, starting with light pressure and gradually changing to heavy. Press once and release, and repeat for one to two minutes. The Laogong acupoint is the acupoint of the Jueyin Pericardium Meridian of Hand (PC), which has the functions of clearing heart fire, removing damp-heat, cooling the blood for calming endogenous wind, regulating *qi* and soothing the stomach, as well as calming the spirit. Frequent massage of the Laogong acupoint can strengthen heart function.

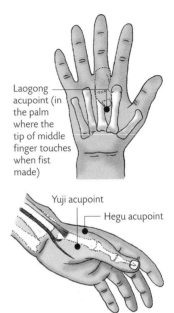

Laogong acupoint (in the palm where the tip of middle finger touches when fist made)

Yuji acupoint

Hegu acupoint

Massage of the Hegu acupoint and Yuji acupoint: This can clear heat and remove dampness, activate the blood and protect the skin, as well as relieve itching and other issues. The Hegu acupoint is the *yuan*-primary point of the Yangming Large Intestine Meridian of Hand (LI) (the point where primordial *qi* enters the body). This can help dredge the movement of *qi* and blood in the surrounding area. The Hegu acupoint is located in the depression between the first and the second metacarpal bones, at the fleshy point where your index finger meets your thumb on the back of your hand. The Yuji acupoint is located at the red and white flesh border of the first metacarpal bone, on the palm, and between the bottom of the thumb and the wrist. The Yangming meridian is full of *qi* and blood, and the Hegu acupoint has the function of activating the blood, regulating *qi*, clearing heat and removing dampness. The Yuji acupoint is an acupoint on the Taiyin Lung Meridian of Hand (LU). The lung is the body's source of water. Therefore, the Yuji acupoint can also clear damp-heat.

Colds

According to traditional Chinese medicine, summer is the season with the most *yang qi*. The weather is hot and full of life, and the metabolism of the human body is at its most vigorous. The body's *yang qi* is external, while *yin* is internal. The circulation of *qi* and blood is also correspondingly vigorous and active on the surface of the body. In order to adapt to the hot climate, the pores of the skin open and release sweat. This helps regulate body temperature, but this at the same time provides a gateway for external assault by wind-cold. The heat in summer also often pushes people to take various measures to prevent heatstroke, such as sitting down, lying flat or sleeping in open places, perhaps in the shade. Many sit under or near electric fans for extended periods, but doing so puts you close to cold air flows, which hurts your *yang qi*. Therefore, in summer, as well as avoiding the summer-heat and dampness, you must be mindful of also avoiding the cold.

Summertime colds often occur after someone suffers from heatstroke during the day, then catches a chill at night. They can result in fever, dizziness, headache, difficulty sweating and body aches and pains. Huoxiang Zhengqi Soft Capsules can be used for treatment. Prevention methods depend mainly on the individual, and on place and time. In summer, you must rest when you are tired and not overwork yourself. It's also a good idea to eat less seafood, and avoid direct blowing of AC or electric fan all night when you sleep. You should also ensure you sleep long enough to maintain your body's natural immune responses. If you do catch a summer cold, your diet should include things like mung bean and lily congee and lotus leaf and wax gourd soup to help you recover.

To prevent colds in summer, the following five things should be done:

Avoid sudden shifts between cold and hot environments. Generally, a difference of about 4 ℃ between the outside and inside temperatures is most appropriate. When entering your home from outside, it is best to go via a non-air-conditioned room first before entering the cooler rooms.

Prioritize sleep. Hot weather burns more energy, and a lack of sleep will accelerate damage to your immune system, making you easily susceptible to illness.

Drink enough water. Water helps the body digest and absorb nutrients, converts food into energy, and strengthens immunity. Water also helps the body cleanse itself of toxins.

Avoid excessive intake of refined sugar and other sweets. Excessive intake of refined white sugar and polysaccharides will lead to "burnout" of the immune system, and diseases will take advantage of this.

Reduce stress and maintain a positive attitude. Adverse psychological tendencies such as pessimism and depression have a real effect. They can lead to an increase in the release of hormones such as cortisol, which directly inhibit the immune system.

Keeping Your Feet Warm

In the hot summer, many people want to cool down. They like to sleep with the windows open at night, especially facing the window with their feet in the cool breeze for comfort. However, this can be very damaging to your health.

Although the bottom of the human feet accounts for just 3.5% of the total body area, it is a highly sensitive area with many nerve endings, acupoints and meridians. This means it is highly sensitive to external stimuli. At night, when the human body is in a deep sleep state, all organs of the body are in a relaxed and natural state, and the feet with their relatively poor resistance to cold can be easily attacked and stimulated by cold and moisture. This directly leads to disorder in the meridian system, causing the body's immune function to decline, which in turn can lead to diseases and frequent colds.

You should not let your body suffer unnecessary damage because you want to keep your feet cool at night. If you find the time, foot massage can be extremely helpful for invigorating the spleen and dispersing stagnated liver-energy, helping clear heat and promote diuresis and enhancing the function of the feet and the whole body. This helps prevent the invasion of moisture, promoting overall health.

2. Exercise for Summer

Many people have a misconception that in summer they should do less, because they don't want to sweat. In fact, it is still necessary to maintain a moderate amount of exercise in summer; just not when the sun is at its peak. Since you sweat more in summer, the key thing to remember is to replace fluids. Drinking enough water helps keep your blood thin.

Sweating can play a role in detoxification, but it is important not to overdo it. This book advises exercising up to a light sweat, then stopping there, to avoid damaging heart *yin*. Summer is a great time for outdoor sports. Effective exercise can improve both blood and *qi* flows, harmonizing *yin* and *yang* in the blood of females. It helps blood merge, dredging the blood vessels and promoting metabolism, aiding the body's natural detoxification systems, which is good for the skin. Because of the heat, it is recommended to exercise in the morning or evening in summer rather than in the middle of the day. Even just taking a walk outside is a form of fitness work, as are more intense forms of exercise such as faster walking, jogging, swimming, yoga, aerobics, and so on.

Precautions for Summer Exercise

During the summer, people are more prone to heatstroke. Heatstroke occurs when body temperature rises sharply and this heat cannot be dissipated quickly enough through sweating. Headaches, dizziness, restlessness and other painful symptoms follow. If the humidity is high, heatstroke is more likely to occur. Therefore, exercise in summer must start from an easy level, and be built up over time so that the body can slowly adapt to the hot weather. You should avoid staying out in the sun for too long, and always stay hydrated.

However, do not gulp down large quantities of cold drinks all at once. During physical exercise, intense muscle use causes the redistribution of blood in the body. A large amount of blood flows to the target muscles and the surface of the body, while the digestive organs lose some blood supply. For this reason, large quantities of ice-cold drinks over-stimulate the stomach, which is already in a vulnerable state. It has insufficient gastric acid concentration, so ice-cold drinks will easily damage its physiological function. If you drink a large amount of cold drinks after physical exercise in summer, issues can range from mild (loss of appetite) to severe (acute gastritis, chronic gastritis, gastric ulcers and other diseases).

Avoid exercising in strong sunlight. Staying out too long in strong sunlight in summer can have very negative effects on your body. The sun's rays contain infrared light, which is particularly strong in the summer. It radiates into the meninges and brain cells through your hair, skin and skull, and too much of this can cause brain lesions and also lead to symptoms similar to heatstroke. For this reason, it is best to do all physical exercise in summer either in the morning or after four o'clock in the afternoon. You should not stay out for too long, or overwork yourself.

Pay attention to skin care. High temperatures and the hot sun in summer can really harm the skin over time. Make sure you thoroughly bathe frequently and wash your face with appropriate skincare products to reduce irritation. It is also crucial to select the right sunscreen for your skin type, and of course, to avoid spending too much time doing sports or other activities in the hot sun.

Choose the right exercise. In the scorching sun of summer, some types of sports are simply not suitable. Consider changing your exercise if the sun is too hot. For example, you might climb stairs instead of hiking on open mountains; walk in the morning and evening instead of running; do indoor activities instead of outdoor football, and so on. One of the most typical summer exercises is swimming, because it is a fun way to stay cool. However, it is not a good idea to go swimming immediately after sweating a lot. Swimming in open water can lead to red-eye diseases, otitis, sinusitis, and various kinds of dermatitis. Make sure you do not swim in polluted or unsafe waters.

Don't take a cold shower immediately after exercise. People often sweat heavily in summer during physical exercise. Some people like to take a cold shower immediately after they exercise, as a form of relief. However, doing so is actually harmful to your health. During physical exercise, your metabolism goes into overdrive, generating a large amount of heat. The capillaries of the skin expand greatly, so as to facilitate heat emission. If you take a cold shower immediately after physical exercise, the skin is stimulated by a harsh drop in temperature, resulting in a sudden contraction of capillaries, which is not conducive to the distribution of body heat. Although you immediately feel cooler, longer term, it becomes uncomfortable. At the same time, sudden cold stimulation will suddenly close the sweat pores that have opened on the body surface, which can easily make you ill.

Looking After Your Neck

Hot weather often means we hardly think about keeping our necks warm. This means that there is an increased risk of neck aches and pains. There are several ways to prevent this:

Avoid bowing your head for long periods of time: Those who have to or tend to hunch their heads forward while working should take a rest every 20 minutes, raising their heads and moving their necks. As a template, perform head raises, chest raises and arm extensions every one to two hours, for about ten minutes.

Reverse extension exercise: Lie on your front and stretch the head, hands and legs back for ten minutes each time, one to two times a day.

Head raise movement: Take a sitting or standing position, cross your hands, put them on the back of your occipital, and repeatedly raise your head with your neck. Your hands will provide resistance. Take a short break and repeat a total of six to eight times. This can also be simplified to a simple resistance-free head extension.

Head rotations: Take a sitting or standing position, hold your hands on the occipital behind your head, clamp your forearms to your temples and rotate your head and neck to either side. Your forearms will provide resistance. After holding for a moment, repeat, alternating left and right, six to eight times each.

The 10:10 trick: At 10:10, the hour hand and minute hand of a clock are nearly symmetrical. Stand or sit upright, raise your arms in the shape of "10:10," lift your chest and inhale deeply. This helps relieve pressure on your neck and upper vertebra.

Chest expansion movement: There are three main types of chest expansion. The first is bending the arm upward in an arc, touching the fingers to the shoulders, and rotating several times clockwise and counterclockwise. The second is bending the arm and moving back and forth from the front of the chest to the back of the shoulder blade. The third is crossing your arms and turning your chest left and right.

Neck self-massage: Self-massage can improve local blood circulation, relieve soft tissue tension, eliminate neck muscle fatigue, and prevent neck stiffness. Common neck self-massage techniques are as follows:

① Press on the Fengchi acupoints with both thumbs for one to two minutes.

② Use the thumb and forefinger of your left or right hand to pinch the muscles on both sides of the cervical spine from behind the neck, or use your thumbs to knead the muscles on both sides of the cervical spine for two to three minutes. Focus on kneading or

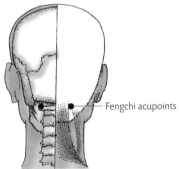

Fengchi acupoints

rubbing the aching points.

③ Place the left hand on the upper part of the right shoulder through the front, and knead or rub the upper part of the supraspinatus with your finger for two to three minutes. Then firmly tap on the supraspinatus with your palm ten times. Massage the left upper shoulder with the right hand in the same way.

Swimming

Swimming is a fantastic, full-body exercise that is useful for many types of sports. Cool water temperature can also be refreshing in summer, making people feel relaxed and happy, and enhancing the body's ability to respond to the outside world. Over time, the body's ability to resist cold and disease is also improved by swimming.

Because of the relative thickness of water compared to air and differences in gravity, the resistance to body movement in the water is 12 times greater than that on land, and staying afloat requires the coordination of all muscles. Swimming can thus comprehensively enhance the function of muscles, joints and bones. In addition to exercising the arms, legs, and abdomen of the human body, it also benefits the internal organs, such as heart, brain, lungs and liver. Swimming is also especially beneficial to the blood vessels, and is sometimes known as "vascular gymnastics." Additionally, because heat is transferred faster through water than through air, people lose heat faster in water than on land. Swimming thus consumes a lot of heat, which means people can easily burn energy and lose weight, if their goal is to do so.

The best time for summer swimming is about 6 am, but swimming from 4 to 5 pm, or after 7 to 8 pm is also a good choice. You should swim for ten minutes to half an hour each time, two to three times a week. The water temperature in summer is lower in the mornings. Before entering the water, wipe yourself with cold water to make sure your body has time to adapt to the cold. This helps prevent cramps.

Jumping

Jumping or bouncing around can strengthen blood circulation and make blood flow to the brain better, providing more oxygen to the brain. At the same time, any jumping or bouncing motion promotes the vitality of various neurotransmitters in the brain, making brain activities more agile. Counting your jumps can encourage brain activity and the tendency to think positively, helping you think faster and make more accurate judgments. Older people in China often do gentle jumping or bouncing exercises, and this has been shown to significantly reduce mental decline, reducing the risk of age-related brain diseases such as Alzheimer's or dementia.

Gymnastics

Aerobics and gymnastics exercises help strengthen balance and coordination, and have obvious effects on muscle building. Here is one balance exercise you might try. Straighten your hands forward, keeping your palms close to the wall and your whole body in a straight line. Bend your elbows, and move your whole body forward and backward, eight to ten times a day. You will benefit if you persevere.

Table Tennis (*Ping-Pong*)

The main cause of myopia is eye fatigue. When playing table tennis, the ciliary muscle relaxes and contracts constantly as you follow the ball. This effortlessly promotes better blood supply to the eye tissue, thus eliminating or reducing eye fatigue, effectively improving vision, and preventing myopia.

3. Leisure in Summer

What recreational activities can help us pass the long hot summer? Try the following two activities for an easygoing, fun and healthy summer.

Fishing

Fishing is not only about catching fish, but also about relaxing and having an enjoyable time. Sitting under the luxuriant shade of trees by a lake or pond, enjoying the feeling of a summer breeze on your skin and listening to the songs of the cicadas at dusk ... It's hard not to let this put you in a good mood. Fishing is a great way to naturally feel relaxed, refreshed, and less irritable or depressed. Frequent experience of this kind of happiness is naturally conducive to health and longevity.

The reason why fishing feels so good for the soul is that it combines the use of your mind, hands and eyes. It's a perfect mix of peacefulness, mindfulness and physical activity. When fishing, the eyes, brain and mind focus on the movement of the rod and line. Most people stay silent, with their mental focus on their elixir field (3 cun below the navel) and physical focus on the static shape in front of them. This stillness directly improves your ability to focus, visually and mentally.

Traveling

Many people like to use the summer to go traveling. One main purpose of summer travel is to gain some relief from the heat, so the healthiest tourist sites to choose are seaside and mountain areas. There are two reasons for this:

First of all, the temperature found in both these two locations tends to be relatively low. Coastal climates, also known as marine climates, are cooler in summer compared to inland. Mountain climates are also characterized by low temperature, and a large temperature difference between day and night. Generally speaking, temperature is inversely proportional to altitude. For every 1000 m increase in altitude, the temperature will drop by 5–6 °C.

Coastal and mountainous areas are also generally pleasant areas to be in. People who live by the sea often find that the wind direction changes regularly throughout both the day and night. Especially on hot summer days, a cool sea breeze on your face is a wonderfully refreshing feeling. Wide, sandy beaches are also a restful and relaxing place to sunbathe and take dips in the sea. Favorable weather conditions in coastal locations help coordinate the functions of various tissues and organs of the body. As a result, staying by the sea has been shown to have a genuine effect on the prevention and treatment of many chronic diseases. A good summer vacation would be to go somewhere by the sea for about ten days, to reap the benefits to your physical and mental health. There are also many benefits of going to the mountains. Generally speaking, the altitude range most beneficial to human health is mid- to low-altitude mountains, that is, with a height of 500 to 2000 meters. This height has a positive effect on human health, mainly reflected in the convalescence of mountain climate and some longevity factors of being in a mountain environment.

4. What to Eat in Summer

In summer, the weather is hot, and plants and animals are actively growing and reproducing. Summer is also the period when bacteria and viruses grow and reproduce fastest. The heat can also affect people's appetite and digestion, reducing the stomach's ability to deal with things. It's a common season for gastrointestinal diseases, such as acute enteritis or diarrhea. So, it's important to be mindful of food hygiene in summer, and protect our health by eating the right things.

The general principles of deciding what to eat in summer are: ① Ensure the foods you eat are mostly light; ② Make sure you're getting enough vitamins; ③ Make sure you're getting enough inorganic salt; ④ Make sure you're getting enough protein.

What Not to Eat

Because of the hot weather, many people think it's a good idea to drink cold drinks in summer. However, traditional Chinese medicine theory believes that eating too many raw, cold products will damage the body's *yang qi*. As the temperature rises, people often experience a loss of appetite. At this time of year, the spleen and stomach are often functioning sluggishly, while the pores of the skin are open and releasing more sweat. This means it is a good time to supplement the diet with plenty of cool, sour and salty flavors. Sour foods not only prevent excessive sweating, but also tempt the appetite in addition to clearing fire and dissipating heat. On the opposite side of the scale, hot-natured fruits such as lychee, mango, pineapple and others can easily lead to excessive internal heat and should be avoided.

A good summer diet includes plenty of light flavors and whole grains to balance this out. Eat fewer foods of a spicy, hot, and dry nature, to avoid harboring too much heat in the body. Avoid fatty, sweet and thick flavors, as this helps avoid internal wind caused by heat accumulation and the development of boils. Always avoid overeating. Food goes off faster in summer, so try not to eat food that is more than a day old. It is a good idea to drink plenty of chrysanthemum tea, mulberry leaf tea, lotus leaf tea and similar foodstuffs which have cooling and anti-heat functions.

Diets Suited to Different Individuals

In daily life, we often see that different people will have different reactions when eating the same food. For example, some people are completely comfortable drinking cold drinks in winter, as if there is heat in the body that has finally been cleared away. Others can't enjoy cold drinks even on hot days, and will experience stomach pain or even diarrhea when ingesting ice-cold beverages. This is because of individual differences in constitution. The constitution of these two groups of people belongs to the "imbalance of *yin* and *yang*."

It is obvious that people who like to drink cold drinks in winter have a hot constitution, that is, strong *yang*. In summer, they are represented by the fire element and thriving *yang* energy. People who prefer cold food are drawn to do so because they aim to clear internal fire and nourish their hearts.

Conversely, those who dislike drinking cold drinks even in summer tend to have cold constitutions, that is, partial *yang* deficiency. People with this constitution should fill their diet with warm and hot foods, to warm the stomach and strengthen the spleen. People who have a strong *yang* constitution and hyperactivity of fire due to *yin* deficiency have a strong basic metabolic rate. These two types of people should eat plenty of cold and cool foods to restrict the internal heat of the body. People with *yang*-deficient constitutions have low basal metabolic rates and less heat generated in their body. Such people should choose more warm foods in their diet to supplement the body's *yang qi*.

Of course, most people have a basic balance of *yin* and *yang*, known as "neutral" in traditional Chinese medicine. As long as they follow the rules of summer diet, this will be maintained. However, the *yin* and *yang* of the human body are always in a state of flux, and balance is maintained within a range. Changes to a person's environment, work, age and so on can all have an effect on them. For example, some women tend to have a *yang* deficiency when they are young, being drawn to heat and fearing the cold, but then may change into a *yin*-deficient constitution when they are menopausal. At this time, they need to adjust their diet according to their body changes, so as to achieve a new balance between *yin* and *yang*.

Water

Drinks such as soda, juice and coca cola contain lots of sugars and electrolytes. These substances will cause adverse stimulation to the stomach, affecting digestion and appetite and increasing the burden of kidney filtration. They can affect kidney function if consumed in large quantities. Eating too much sugar can fill the body with excess energy, leading to unhealthy weight gain. Therefore, it is not advisable to drink non-water beverages in summer. It is better to drink water as much as you can, especially for children and the elderly.

In summer, when you sweat a lot, fluid loss is a serious concern. You must replace your fluids, but you must also do it in the correct way. If you drink too much water in one go, this may lead to a decrease in the concentration of salt in the blood, putting your urination system into overdrive and resulting in water shortage in the body and dehydration symptoms. It's always better to replenish water in small amounts. Drink water every 20 to 30 minutes, in regular amounts, to help slow down the body's sweat rate and reduce water loss. When sweating heavily, it is also a good idea to drink beverages high in electrolytes (such as slightly salted water or sports drinks) to supplement the lost salt. Don't wait until you are thirsty to drink, and don't drink too much when you are thirsty. Do not drink a lot of water before going to bed or when eating.

Sodium

How much sodium (salt) you need to eat depends on how much you sweat. Over an eight-hour work day, you should sweat out no more than four liters, and you should ensure you're getting 18 grams of salt from your daily diet. If you sweat more than six liters, you need to supplement your sodium intake via electrolyte drinks.

Vitamins

In summer, the body's vitamin requirements are one to two times higher than normal. Large doses of vitamin B1, vitamin B2, vitamin C, vitamin A, vitamin E, etc. have a certain effect on improving heat resistance and physical strength. Vitamin C is found in large amounts in tomatoes, watermelons, melons, peaches, plums and other foods. B vitamins are more abundant in grains, beans, animal liver, lean meat and eggs.

Vinegar

When it's hot outside and you're sweating a lot, consuming more vinegar can increase the concentration of gastric acid in the stomach, aiding digestion and increasing appetite. Vinegar also has strong antibacterial qualities, helping kill off food-poisoning pathogens, such as staphylococcus. It can help protect against intestinal infectious diseases such as typhoid and dysentery. In summer, people are prone to fatigue, drowsiness, and general discomfort. A little vinegar in the diet can quickly relieve fatigue and maintain plenty of energy.

Hot Tea

Drinks are indispensable in summer. However, your first choice should not in fact be something ice cold, or a coffee, but simply hot tea. Tea is rich in potassium, which can quench thirst and ease fatigue. According to expert tests, the cooling capacity of hot tea is actually much greater than that of cold drinks, making it one of the best things to drink in summer to cool down.

Potassium Supplements

In summer, as the temperature continues to rise, our sweat is also losing a lot, especially when working or exercising in high temperature environments. In addition to water and sodium, sweat also contains a certain amount of potassium ions. If the human body sweats a lot in summer, the potassium ions will be lost, which can lead to potassium deficiency in the body.

Potassium is an indispensable mineral in the human body. Its main function in the human body is to maintain the acid-base balance and the normal function of nerve muscles. A lack of potassium in the body can cause neuromuscular weakness and lethargy. In addition, serious potassium deficiency can lead to decreased heart function, decreased blood supply to the brain, dizziness, fatigue and weakness.

In summer, prevention is better than cure. Make sure you're eating enough potassium-rich foods in your daily diet. Eat plenty of fruits, vegetables, beans or bean products, kelp, eggs, etc. that have high potassium content.

In fresh vegetables, the potassium content of fungi (such as button mushrooms, fresh mushrooms, etc.), long beans, cauliflower, pumpkin, rape, spinach, celery, etc. is particularly high. Among fruits, banana has the highest potassium content. In addition, seasonal summer fruits such as cherries, apricots, lychees and strawberries are also rich in potassium. Seafood is also an important source of potassium, including foods such as kelp, seaweed, sea fish, shrimp, etc.

A healthy summer diet also includes nuts, such as peanuts, walnuts and pistachios, to supplement the lost potassium. In addition, you can also drink mung bean soup. This helps prevent heatstroke and cools down the body, and can also help supplement your potassium intake.

After sweating a lot, your body needs potassium and sodium ions. Drinks are a good way to get these nutrients in, but do not drink too much water or large amounts of sugary drinks immediately, as this can actually reduce your levels of blood potassium.

Heatstroke Prevention Soups and Congees

① Shredded Pork with Towel Gourd and Balsam Pear Soup

Ingredients: 250 g fresh towel gourd, 250 g fresh balsam pear (pulp removed), 200 g lean pork

Method: Slice the towel gourd and balsam pear and shred the lean pork, putting them all into a soup pot. Add one liter of water to cook, and then salt to taste.

Effects: Clears heat and detoxifies; replenishes deficiencies. It can relieve excessive body heat, thirst, dizziness, and sore throat.

② Yam Soup

Ingredients: 100 g Chinese yam, 100 g pork tenderloin

Method: First peel and wash the yam and shred it with the pork. Put both into a soup pot, and add appropriate amount of boiling water and boil until the meat is cooked. Season with salt to taste.

Effects: Helps replenish spleen *qi*, nourish *yin* and relieve heat. Helps relieve symptoms such as dizziness, lack of appetite, fatigue, thirst and excessive drinking.

③ Lotus Seed Soup

Ingredients: 20 g lotus seeds, 10 g coix seeds, 10 g gordon euryale seeds, 6 g dried tremella (reconstituted)

Method: Fry the first three ingredients together in a pot. Then add some water and tremella, and stew them together until a soup is made.

Effects: Invigorates the spleen and stops diarrhea, eliminating dampness and facilitating diuresis. This product can relieve symptoms such as diarrhea, lack of appetite and urination (due to excessive sweating).

④ Sour Plum Soup

Ingredients: 25 g hawthorn berries, 25 g black plums, 5 g liquorice roots, 5 g osmanthus

Method: Combine all the above ingredients into a soup, and then season with rock sugar to taste.

Effects: Relieves heat and aids digestion, detoxifying and beautifying. Black plums also have an anti-allergic effect, and have a good prevention and treatment effect on minor acne flare-ups and spots caused by skin allergies.

⑤ Pear Congee

Ingredients: three pears, rice as desired

Method: Wash and chop three pears, add some water, boil for half an hour, remove the pear dregs, add rice, boil them into congee, and eat them while hot.

Effects: Clears internal heat and relieves cough symptoms, moistens the lungs and aids digestion. Eating this soup while it is hot can cure wind-heat in children, lung-heat cough, loss of appetite, and dizziness.

⑥ Congee with Watermelon Peel

Ingredients: 250 g watermelon peel (remove the hard rind and residual pulp), 100 g japonica rice

Method: Cut the watermelon peel into small pieces and marinate it with salt. Take the pot and put the watermelon peel in it with water, and the washed japonica rice. Boil both on high heat first, then simmer them for about 15 minutes. Season to taste with salt.

Effects: Helps eliminate internal heat, relieves heatstroke, encourages clear fluid production and quenches thirst, induces diuresis to reduce edema. It is used to treat internal heat and thirst, heatstroke and dizziness, short and brown urine, nephritis and edema, diabetes, etc.

5. Summer Lifestyle

In the heat of summer, do you always find yourself looking for a way to keep cool? Do you struggle to do so, no matter what you're doing? Unexpectedly, many of the most habitual ways people keep themselves cool are actually harmful. Summer is the season of high energy consumption. If you don't pay attention to health maintenance at this time, your physique will decline and your resistance will weaken in autumn and winter, which will affect your health throughout the year. So, how do we change the season of summer from one of burning energy to one of restoring energy? The key is to follow the laws of summer and live scientifically to preserve one's health.

Four Things to Avoid

It is hot in summer, and many people like to drink tea in the shade to relieve the heat. However, it should be noted that in summer, the body's *yang qi* is flowing on the outside, and is weak inside of the body. There are four things we should avoid in summer in order to preserve health:

Avoid drinking tea on an empty stomach. Drinking a lot of tea, especially on an empty stomach, can easily lead to the depletion of *yang qi*. If you are a person who likes salty food, food that is savory in nature promotes tea to be drawn towards the kidney. This reduces kidney *yang* of the lower *jiao*, making people prone to arthralgia syndrome, that is, hand and foot pain, as well as diarrhea, impotence, dysmenorrhea and other diseases caused by the coldness and deficiency of original *qi* of the lower *jiao.* Therefore, it is advisable to drink only two to three cups of tea after meals in summer, and stop drinking immediately if you feel hungry.

Avoid bathing in cold water. Cold water baths or showers are used by many young or middle-aged men to stop themselves from overheating, but in summer, everyone's sweat pores are wide open. To use a small analogy, a sweat gland or pore is like a door. In summer, when the door is open, cold air and wind pathogens can easily enter, causing a serious loss of *yang*. Visible symptoms of this include cold hands and feet, spasm of calf, blurred vision, and even heat syndrome that can appear without cause. At the same time, even if you take a hot bath, you should also pay attention to avoiding cold air flow after you get out. This is especially the case for children.

Avoid sleeping with the AC on. It is not advisable to turn on the air conditioner all night when sleeping. This can easily lead to colds, facial paralysis, joint pain, abdominal pain and diarrhea, seriously damaging the body. For children, do not fan them to cool them down after they fall asleep, or they can easily start to suffer from hand and foot convulsions, an inability to open their mouth, rheumatism and other diseases. However, it is so hot in summer that it is often unrealistic to refuse to turn on the air conditioner at all. So, AC should be used with a few rules: ① Do not stand directly in front of the air coming out, and do not allow the cold air to flow onto your abdomen, head or the soles of your feet; ② Generally, the air setting should be gentle, especially for children. Do not set it to circulate air too fast or too hard; ③ The air flow should be time-controlled, and the settings appropriately reduced when the room feels less hot.

Avoid eating raw, cold foods at night. In summer when the nights are shorter, those who are slightly weaker or older often have cold stomachs, and find it less easy to digest food. Lettuce, melons and other raw, cold foodstuffs should not be eaten at night. In addition, do not eat meat, noodles, or greasy foods at night, or you may have abdominal distension and other symptoms.

Sleeping Late, Rising Early

Summer nights are often hot and humid, and many people find it difficult to sleep well. Tossing and turning all night can be very uncomfortable. A lack of sleep often has an impact on your mood the next day. In fact, summer is characterized by long days and short nights. People go to bed later and get up earlier, and the hours you sleep are naturally meant to be shorter. This is in line with the principle of being in harmony with nature. Chinese medicine experts believe that when it is too hot to fall asleep easily, it's a good idea to sleep half an hour later than usual. In the morning, you should still get up at the usual time, or even half an hour earlier, and this will have absolutely no impact on your health. Just be careful not to sleep later than midnight. It is not a good idea to sleep later than this, or stay up all night. If you do not sleep at the appropriate time, when you are tired, it will be very difficult to fall asleep later on, and you may be unable to sleep at all.

Taking Naps

In summer, the days are long and the nights are short. The temperature is high and the human body's metabolism is working well. Energy consumption is high, and fatigue comes quickly. In addition, it is hot at night and sleep is prone to be disturbed, resulting in insufficient sleep. Many people find that taking a nap at noon in summer can have a good effect on their overall sleeping habits. Naps help rest all systems of the body, and are a good way to replenish energy in the afternoon. Napping is also a good measure to prevent heatstroke. Note, however, that it is not appropriate to take a nap immediately after lunch. A better method is to do some light activity after lunch, such as walking or rubbing the abdomen, and then take a nap. This is conducive to the digestion and absorption of food. Afternoon naps should last 30 to 50 minutes, and no more than one hour. Too long a nap will not only affect your sleep at night, but make you drowsy and dull after waking up, which is counterproductive.

Staying Away from Air Vents

In summer, there are often people who are greedy for coolness at night, and turn their AC down too low with the vent blowing onto their faces. The next morning, they find their mouth cannot close, and they cannot drink water without spilling anything, or speak clearly. This is because the AC brings down their resistance and damages facial nerves, especially on a hot day.

Don't rush straight to the AC on a hot day, and do not fall victim to the temptation of putting electric fans close to your face. If you are treating any kind of sickness, it is crucial to avoid being exposed to wind and cold pathogens, including those that come from electric fans or AC. Hot compresses can be applied locally on the face; you should drink plenty of water, eat light, tasteless flavor foods, and avoid spicy food.

Protecting the Upper Body

Since summer is so hot, many people like to wear crop tops that expose the stomach. Some people also like to sleep with their upper body naked. Neither of these is good for your health. In summer, the heat produced by the body is higher than the temperature outside the body, and the skin and muscle microvessels are in a state of relaxation, especially during sleep. The nervous system is less sensitive to stimuli, which puts the whole body in a basically "defenseless" state, so wind pathogens can easily invade. So, in summer, you should wear clothes to sleep at night, and you must not expose your chest or back. Even if you feel it's unbearable hot, you should still always protect your abdomen to prevent wind pathogens from invading the body and skin, and finding their way into your internal organs. In addition, after sweating a lot in summer, you should change your clothes as soon as possible. Do not let them dry on your body. Otherwise, not only will your *yang qi* be damaged, but moisture will also enter the body to heat up, which causes damp-heat syndrome and leads to skin diseases such as sores or rheumatism.

Skin Rescue

If your skin is sunburned: In summer, the sun is powerful and can burn you. If the skin on your face and body is sunburned, what should you do? If you get sunburned, you should apply a cotton pad dipped in soothing toner to your face. It is best to apply it alternately until your skin feels cool again. After this, slowly dab the cold pad on the rest of your face, nose and other red skin patches. You might also use some ice. After this, use moisturizer.

First aid for skin burns: When the skin is burned by strong sunlight and feels extremely hot, put toner into the refrigerator to cool, and then apply frozen. If it's available, you might also use a moisture-rich mask.

First aid if the skin feels painful: When the skin feels tender, it has almost reached the point of scalding. The only first aid is to apply ice compresses instead of applying any skincare products. If the hands and feet are sunburned, wrap a block of ice with a towel soaked in water and apply until the skin feels soothed.

When the sunburned skin feels a little soothed, to prevent the skin from feeling dry and tight, or even cracking, you should simply try to rehydrate. First, use a foaming face cream to moisturize when bathing, and then rinse off after a period of time. Then, apply the lotion containing moisturizing ingredients on the face, and gently press the face with the palm of your hand to promote the skin's absorption of moisture. After doing this several times, the skin will restore its original moisturizing ability.

6. Emotional Health in Summer

In summer, the weather is hot and everyone is sweating more than before. Traditional Chinese medicine believes that "sweat is the liquid of the heart." and a large amount of fluid loss also leads to a loss of *qi*. This can damage the heart. Damage to the *qi* and *yin* of the heart can be expressed in people feeling upset and impatient, resulting in a decline in productivity and efficiency at work or in school.

Therefore, in the heat of summer, it's important to adjust our spirit. We need to find ways to keep our moods steady. As a Chinese saying goes, "You will cool off as you calm down." Keeping our mood calm helps us to make sure we spend our summer peacefully and happily.

Emotional Outlets

The method of using given actions or rituals to relieve unpleasant emotional reactions is known as using emotional outlets. For example, many people use hobbies to channel their emotions, such as music, chess, calligraphy or painting. Healthcare experts believe that "for patients suffering from any of the seven emotions, reading books and listening to music to relieve depression often has better results than taking medicine." Physical outlets may also be used. Health care experts believe that when you are overthinking and in a bad mood, you should go out traveling or for exercise, allowing the scenery to regulate negative emotions. Many people find that being amongst nature helps you to relax and relieves worry.

Transcending Emotions

Using reason can also help overcome the interference of bad emotions. Some find that they can "turn grief into strength," and through training their mind, learn to turn unpleasant stimuli, such as physical and mental pain, into vigorous and positive action.

Explaining Emotions

Relieving the mental worries of patients by means of explanation, encouragement, consolation and exhortation, improving their confidence in overcoming the pain, so as to cooperate with treatment and promote rehabilitation.

Reducing Emotions

By moderating and harmonizing emotions, we can prevent the seven emotions from being excessive, so as to achieve the goal of psychological balance.

Venting Emotions

In life, people spend more time in adversity than in prosperity. When they are in adversity, depressed and scared, they should learn to not restrain the negative emotion, but to vent it. There are many ways to relieve stress. One might find friends to chat to; or emotions can be vented into a single argument, or by allowing oneself to weep.

7. Physiotherapy and Health in Summer

Summer fatigue makes many people sitting in an office miserable. According to traditional Chinese medicine, sleepiness in summer is mainly related to heat and humidity. During the long summers, the humidity is heavy. The spleen is the organ that responds most to humidity, and in humid weather, it creates a fatigue response. This can be relieved by massaging the Baihui acupoint, Taiyang acupoints, and Fengchi acupoints. Various "high temperature diseases" can strike in summer. Pressing on the Taichong, Shaochong, Zhongchong and Guanchong acupoints can help reduce the risk of these diseases, allowing you to properly enjoy your summer.

Massaging the Taiyang Acupoints

The Taiyang acupoints are located at the midpoint of the line between the eyebrow tip and the outer corner of the eye, about one finger width backward. Massaging this point can not only refresh your spirit, but also relieve headaches. When massaging, place your thumbs or forefinger on the Taiyang acupoint on both sides respectively, and gently rotate in a circular motion for 30 seconds. Anyone can use this method, be sure you do not press too hard. Massage with moderate force until you feel slight soreness in the acuopoint. How often you do this is an individual choice. Frequency can be adjusted according to the degree of fatigue.

Massaging the Baihui Acupoint

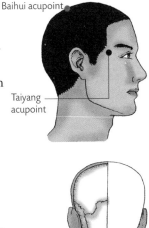

The Baihui acupoint is located at the highest point in the middle of the head. Massaging here can refresh the spirit and stimulate the flow of *yang qi*. When massaging, press both of your thumbs or forefingers on the acupoint, slowly and forcefully, until you feel slightly sore, and press for 30 seconds. At the same time, you can do gentle circular massage five times.

Massaging the Fengchi Acupoints

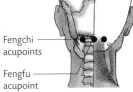

The Fengchi acupoints are located at the neck, under the occipital bone, and at the same level as the Fengfu acupoint (at the center of the back hairline, 1 cun up). In addition to refreshing, this type of massage can also relieve eye fatigue, and is especially useful for those who work in front of a computer or at a desk for long periods. When massaging, keep your body upright, and put your thumbs on the Fengchi acupoints. Tilt your head back, rotate your thumbs in a circle and massage the acupoints for one minute, until you can feel a clear soreness. Repeat five times.

Massaging the Taichong Acupoints

The Taichong acupoints are located on the top of both feet, at the rear depression of the first metatarsal space. In midsummer, for complaints of dizziness, thirst, nausea, palpitation, chest tightness or other symptoms of heatstroke, the patient or a family member should press firmly on the acupoint with their thumb. It is better to pinch and press with the fingernail tip, with a certain degree of strength, so that the patient feels a little pain or numbness. Hold for half to one minute, and then press the other foot. Alternatively, press the right Taichong

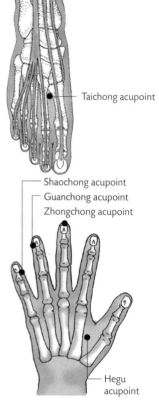

Taichong acupoint

Shaochong acupoint
Guanchong acupoint
Zhongchong acupoint

Hegu acupoint

acupoint with the left thumb for three minutes, and then press the left Taichong acupoint with the right thumb pulp for three minutes. Repeat 2 to 3 times for 10 to 15 minutes. It should be noted that anyone with blood coagulation disorders should be careful when using this technique. Pregnant women should not use it.

Massaging the Zhongchong Acupoints

The Zhongchong acupoints are located in the center of the tip of both middle fingers. When suffering from heatstroke symptoms such as dizziness, thirst, nausea, palpitation, etc., the patient or a family member should press the acupoint with their thumb. It is best to pinch and press it with the fingernail tip, with a certain degree of strength, so that the patient feels a little numbness, or swelling pain. Massage for half a minute to one minute, and then do the other hand.

Massaging the Guanchong Acupoints

The Guanchong acupoints are located at the ulnar side of the end of both ring fingers, 0.1 cun from the root of the nail. When suffering from heatstroke symptoms such as dizziness, headache, giddiness, thirst, nausea and vomiting occur, the patient or a family member should press the acupoint with their thumb. It is best to pinch and press it with the fingernail tip, with a certain degree of strength, until the patient feels some numbness and swelling pain.

Hold for half to one minute, and then do the other hand.

Massaging the Shaochong Acupoints

The Shaochong acupoints are located at the radial side of the
distal segment of both little fingers, 0.1 cun from the nail.
When using this acupoint, the patient should be seated with
their palms down. In the heat of summer, when suffering
from dizziness, thirst, nausea, psychological distress and other
heatstroke symptoms, the patient or a family member should
press the acupoint with their thumb, preferably with the
fingertip, pinching and pressing with a certain degree of strength
so the patient feels a little numbness and swelling pain. Massage
for half a minute to one minute, and then do the other hand.
Alternatively, gently clamp the depression on both sides of the
left pinkie nail with the thumb and forefinger, and gently knead
the acupoint in a vertical direction. It is worth noting that this
acupoint is a reflex area linked to the brain. You should knead
it slowly, and not use brute force. Your left and right hands can
knead one another.

Pressing the Emergency Acupoints

In addition to massaging the above acupoints, you can also take
advantage of several "emergency acupoints" found on the human
body, such as Renzhong, Dazhui, Hegu (see left page), and
Zusanli acupoints. Press and rub them for several minutes for a
heat-relieving, heat-clearing effect.

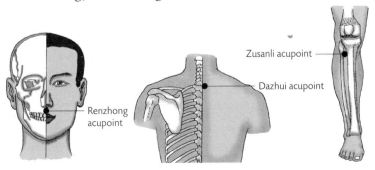

Zusanli acupoint

Dazhui acupoint

Renzhong
acupoint

Chapter Three
Fall

A s fall descends, it brings with it a feeling of relief, as the air begins to finally cool. Autumn breezes rustle through the trees, and rain falls softly on the piles of yellowing leaves. Young and old, male and female, everyone should be thinking about how to keep themselves healthy during the fall.

Fall can be divided into three stages: early, mid and late fall. Each stage of fall has different characteristics, and our health care should reflect them, utilizing slightly different countermeasures to each change in the climate we find ourselves in.

In the early fall period, the heat of midsummer has not quite disappeared, and the weather can still be very hot and humid. In traditional Chinese medicine, the period of late summer and early fall is called the "long summer," and the main *qi* of the long summer's "six climatic exopathogens" is dampness. Therefore, at this time of year, attention should still be paid to heatstroke prevention and cooling, a timely supplement of water, and special attention should be paid to prevent the evil of damp-heat and cold-damp from invading the body.

At mid-autumn, rainfall gradually decreases, the weather gets drier, and the days are hot while the nights are cool. The climate in this period is characterized by "dryness," and dryness pathogens have a high likelihood of hurting the lungs and stomach. Therefore, an important focus of health preservation in the fall is to nourish *yin* energy, which prevents dryness and helps moisten the lungs and stomach. The dry climate means that people's sweat evaporates quickly from their bodies. This often leads to dry skin, increasing the visibility of wrinkles and causing dry mouths and throats, dry coughs, and even hair loss and constipation. Therefore, it is a good approach to try and maintain a certain humidity indoors, and always ensure you are drinking plenty of water. This helps preserve your body's essential *qi* and clear fluid, even during strenuous activity.

As we move into the late fall, winds pick up and the weather cools significantly. Temperatures may drop very suddenly. The cold is on its way, and as it approaches, illnesses such as chronic tracheitis, emphysema, joint pain, and cardiovascular and cerebrovascular diseases become increasingly common. The key in fall is not only to prevent dryness pathogens from hurting the body, but also to prevent the cold pathogen from hurting the body. It's a very good idea to be doing exercise which helps you withstand the cold. However, the elderly and anyone who already has chronic health issues would do better to simply wrap up warm and ensure they don't lose too much body heat. This helps prevent diseases related to cold. It's also very important to keep an eye on our emotions at this time of year, avoiding any negative triggers that weigh down the spirit and working to maintain a positive, calm mindset.

Throughout the three months of fall, *yang qi* gradually subsides and *yin qi* gradually increases its presence. The autumn winds start to pick up, and the weather is getting cooler. Everything in nature has naturally matured and entered its harvest season. Traditional Chinese medicine stresses the interconnectivity of man and nature. Humans, just like plants, are slowly experiencing a gradual decrease of *yang qi* in their bodies. This is why, in the fall, traditional Chinese medicine emphasizes this principle of bodily "harvesting." The human body "sprouts" in spring and summer, just like plants, and in the fall it enters its harvesting and storing season. At this time, the body's material demand for *yin* essence increases. If it gets enough, this provides a strong basis for growth after winter. This is why many TCM health practitioners support the concept of "nourishing *yin* in fall and winter."

1. Prevention in Fall

Fall weather is highly changeable, but it is by nature a cool season. It is this kind of "coolness" involves gradually lowering temperatures, which can often induce or aggravate various diseases, such as asthma, angina pectoris, dyspepsia, biliary colic, embolism, stokes and other diseases. The coolness of fall can lead to fluctuations in people's spirit and mood, which often manifest as fatigue, displeasure, insomnia, dizziness and irritability.

Respiratory Problems

The volatile weather in fall can be difficult for people's bodies to adapt to. The temperature variation between morning and night increases, which means that the mucus found in the human respiratory system is constantly being stimulated by sudden heat and then sudden cold. This weakens resistance, providing an opportunity for pathogenic microorganisms to sneak in and cause respiratory problems like colds, tonsillitis, tracheitis and pneumonia. Immunocompromised people, such as the elderly or children with chronic bronchitis, are very vulnerable to the impact of fall weather, and are more likely to catch weather-related colds and coughs. It is cooler in the morning and evening during fall, making it easier to catch colds. These can in turn induce airway and tracheal problems. The symptoms of patients with chronic bronchitis and asthma are often aggravated at this time of year. Fall is also a peak season for allergic rhinitis. If you experience frequent sneezing, a runny nose, nasal congestion, and nasal itching during fall, they may be caused by this disease. In fall, therefore, it is a good idea to keep an eye on one's respiratory health.

The following methods can be used to prevent colds in autumn:

Cold face washes, hot foot baths: Get into the habit of washing your face with cold water in the morning and soaking your feet with hot water in the evening. Doing this every day helps "prevent colds entering the skin."

Physical fitness: It's especially important in fall and winter to walk and do sports outside. Constant exercise helps improve your body's ability to resist cold, helping you fight sickness.

Drinking ginger tea: Instead of regular tea, brew a good amount of ginger and brown sugar together for an effective cold cure and prevention drink.

Stomach Problems

There are four reasons why people are more prone to gastrointestinal diseases in fall. The first is that, in summer, people tend to lose their appetite because of the high temperature. In fall, the climate cools, meaning people's appetite comes back, and people find themselves eating too much, which leads to diarrhea due to spleen deficiencies. Second, since people spend a lot of time cooling down in the summer, their bodies get used to seeking out coolness. By the time fall rolls around, and this habit has not changed, many people suffer from colds, accompanied by diarrhea and other gastrointestinal symptoms; this is a seasonal phenomenon called cold dysentery. The third reason is that we eat more vegetables in summer and less meat and fish. In fall, we usually eat more meat and fish. If this shift happens too fast, our gastrointestinal tract struggles to cope, resulting in functional allergies called allergic enteritis. The fourth reason is that there are more flies in fall than in summer, and flies are a main vector via which dysentery bacteria are transmitted. It is therefore important to be on the lookout for bacillary dysentery in the fall.

To prevent gastrointestinal problems, first of all, we should pay attention to strengthening the spleen. We can do this by eating more lentils, yams, leeks, radishes and so on, so that even eating large amounts is unlikely to cause diarrhea. This way, even if you slightly get cold, it will not easily cause gastrointestinal symptoms. Another step in prevention of stomach upset is to pay close attention to food and personal hygiene. Never eat with flies around, and do not eat raw or cold food, to avoid food-borne diseases. When eating meat, seasoning with raw garlic or putting extra garlic paste into recipes can help you avoid dysentery bacilli. If you have diarrhea but it is not from a bacterial infection, take the Chinese medicine "Huoxiang Zhengqi Liquid." It is effective in the treatment of digestion problems, including diarrhea, excessive internal heat and seasonal colds. For bacterial stomach infections, purslane with garlic paste is also effective. Attention should also be paid to the sanitation and disinfection of tableware in autumn, and dishwashing cloths should be disinfected at least two to three times a week.

Diarrhea in Young Children

Another common disease in fall is diarrhea in infants and toddlers. These infections are mainly transmitted via the gastrointestinal tract (the stomach). Because infant feces contain a large number of rotavirus particles and are relatively stable, they can very easily leave traces on their surroundings and infect the people within. Another common cause of infection is infant caretakers' unwashed hands, and the contamination of milk bottles, toys and other baby products. Infants and young children with gastrointestinal problems often experience acute symptoms such as diarrhea, abdominal pain, vomiting, and fever. They may have more than ten bowel movements a day, with large volumes of soupy-textured stool. Most children will also experience different degrees of dehydration in this scenario, which can be life-threatening in severe cases. Parents should therefore not deal with the problem blindly, and seek medical advice.

The following points should be paid attention to in case of children's autumn diarrhea: First, do not use antibiotics. Clinical studies have confirmed that antibacterial drugs are ineffective for this disease. Second, do not use antipyretics, because taking antipyretics will cause a lot of sweating and aggravate dehydration. If the body temperature is too high, try to physically cool the body instead. Third, the child should be given small amounts of easily digestible liquid diet, constantly.

If the child is also vomiting, do not force them to eat or drink. Stop giving them anything for several hours, and allow the intestines and stomach to rest. Fourth, always remember that fluid replacement is the key to the treatment of diarrhea.

Disease Caused by Excessive Dryness

In fall, there is less rain and the weather is dry. The human body is prone to "autumn dryness" due to flaring up of deficient fire. According to traditional Chinese medicine, dryness can easily damage the lungs, and autumn *qi* is connected with the lung *qi* in the human body. Lung *qi* that is too strong can easily lead to insufficient body fluid, resulting in what Chinese medicine terms "dryness disease." This expresses as a lack of fluid in the body, and causes coughs, dry lips, dry skin, hair loss, dry stools and other dehydration-related issues. Ensuring you are drinking plenty of water is the best way to prevent this. However, how you drink your water matters. It is best to drink small amounts of water frequently. Remember not to drink too much at once, because doing so increases the burden on your gastrointestinal tract and can cause abdominal discomfort. In addition, it is a good idea to eat foods that moisten the lungs and promote fluid production, nourishing *yin* and relieving internal dryness. These foods include pears, apples, bananas, kiwi and other fruits; polished round-grained rice, millet, coix seed and other grains; cucumber, lotus root, kelp and other vegetables. TCM also advises eating fewer spicy and pungent things, such as chili, scallion, ginger, garlic, etc. It is very important to get into good habits with work-life balance and sleeping patterns, too. Make sure you go to bed on time, and try to get up early.

In fall, many people experience a sore throat and think it is a cold, at which point they instinctively decide to take cold medicine. However, often what they are experiencing is in fact "autumn dryness," which is mainly manifested by a feeling of dryness and heat across the whole body. It causes dry lips and also a certain mental restlessness. Some people may also have mouth sores, a sore throat and other symptoms, and their skin may also be red and spotty. Although "autumn dryness" is not a serious illness, it does reduce immunity, especially in middle-aged and elderly people, and can increase the severity of other problems. Drinking water is not the only thing you should do, either. To combat "autumn dryness," it really is best to cultivate a healthy mindset, diet and exercise regime.

Mindset: Generally, this means staying positive, and doing things that make us feel good such as walking outside, trying new things and breathing the fresh air. This helps harness spirit *qi*, preventing the lungs from being damaged by dryness pathogens.

Diet: Drink plenty of water, and include some porridge in your diet too. Eat more soybean milk, lily bulbs, radish, honey and other lung-moistening foods. Sweet fruits such as pears and sugarcanes are great choices, and secondly, water chestnuts, bananas, and loquats are also good moisturizing foods. You may wish to also take some health supplements, but take care not to consume too much warm- or hot-natured foods and medicines. These foods include meats like mutton, and supplements like ginseng because they can aggravate autumn dryness.

Do plenty of exercise: Sports should be easy and gentle, but not done to excess. Regularly playing sports and engaging in fitness activities in the morning or evening is a good idea in fall. This might include going on long walks, jogging, or other outdoor activities that help boost overall health. Frequent exercise for fall not only helps regulate the heart and lungs and improves the function of internal organs, but also enhances the immune function of various tissues and organs.

Dampness Pathogen

In early fall, the summer-heat has not yet dissipated, and there tends to be a lot of rain. During this time, we need to prevent the dampness and *yin* pathogens from damaging spleen *yang* and causing edema or diarrhea. If the spleen is hurt by dampness in this period of early fall, it will plant the root of diseases in winter, so it is very important to prevent dampness in this period. The main way to do this is to remove dampness and relieve stagnation from your body, and consume things that help harmonize the stomach and spleen, such as lotus seed, coix seed, lotus root, yam, etc.

Cardio-Cerebrovascular Disease

The fall is also a high-incidence season for cardiovascular and cerebrovascular diseases. As the weather turns cool, the blood vessels of the skin and subcutaneous tissue are in a state of contraction, increasing resistance within the blood vessels. This increases cardiovascular load, leading to an increase in blood pressure. In addition, cold weather can also cause coronary artery spasms, directly affecting the blood supply to the heart, and inducing angina pectoris or myocardial infarction. Therefore, anyone with a history of cardiovascular problems should take precautions. You must consume the correct medicine, and do everything you can to prevent colds and maintain a healthy physical exercise regime. This helps strengthen the body's immunity, so as to avoid inducing or aggravating the disease. Middle-aged and elderly people that suffer from high blood pressure (hypertension), hyperlipidemia, diabetes, or who are overweight or obese may experience symptoms such as headaches, toothaches, arthralgia, abdominal pain and vomiting, which should not be ignored. If the symptoms become severe, sufferers should go to a hospital at once for diagnosis and treatment, because these may be signs of acute cardiovascular and cerebrovascular diseases.

Fall Weight Gain

When the weather cools in the fall, we naturally respond by subconsciously eating a little more. We increase our calorie intake; the weather is pleasant and comfortable; we're getting plenty of sleep and sweating less. As winter approaches, it's natural for the body to store a little more fat as a layer of insulation, as it absorbs more energy than it uses. Many factors may lead to your weight gain if you are not careful. Although many people believe that storing a little extra fat for winter is normal, this should not be excessive and not everyone needs it. Middle-aged and elderly people with cardio-cerebrovascular diseases for example should not really be gaining any fat at all.

How to avoid fall weight gain? First, eat more low-calorie diet foods, such as red beans, radishes, coix seeds, kelp, mushrooms, and coarse grains or cereals. Second, increase your energy consumption via physical activity. Autumn is a good season to travel, not only because of the beautiful fall scenery, but also because the temperature is perfect for plenty of outdoor fun. This kind of vacation can help you avoid weight gain.

2. Exercise for Fall

In the fall, the air is fresh and the temperature lovely and cool. After the scorching heat and humidity of summer, people are almost always delighted when fall comes around. This is the perfect season for exercise. The transition from hot to cold that fall represents is also reflected in the shift from *yang* to *yin* energy. The human body also reflects this pattern. Fall is a time for the body to nourish itself internally. Therefore, a good fall exercise regime should also comply with this principle. Don't do too much exercise, to prevent the loss of sweat and the loss of *yang qi*. Traditional Chinese medicine advocates doing low intensity exercises in autumn, such as climbing and light jogging, for this reason.

Precautions for Fall Exercise

Prevention of sport-related injuries: Because the blood vessels will contract reflexively under low temperature, muscle elasticity will be significantly reduced, as will joint flexibility and the nervous system. If you are not fully warmed up before exercise, it is very easy to injure your muscles, tendons, ligaments and joints.

Prevention of chills and colds: The temperature is low

on autumn mornings, so make sure you do not go outside in a single layer. Make sure you warm up and cool down properly before and after exercise. After exercise, take off sweaty clothes as soon as possible and change into dry ones. Do not wear wet clothes in the cold wind to avoid catching a cold.

Don't overdo it: Fall is the stage when the body's *yang qi* converges, so exercise should also comply with this principle. This means that the amount of exercise should not be too large, to prevent excessive sweating and loss of *yin* fluid. Exercise should be easy and gentle, with light activity.

Prevention of dryness: *The Yellow Emperor's Classic of Medicine* lists dryness as the main *qi* feature of fall. Dryness is also the main external pathogen that can hurt the human body in this period. Because the temperature decreases in autumn, the air humidity also decreases, and the human body is prone to accumulate some dry heat, causing symptoms such as dry throat, lack of saliva in the mouth and tongue, dry lips, nose bleeding, dry stool and so on. In addition, the loss of water during exercise will aggravate adverse reactions, and may cause you to be very thirsty or to urinate less than normal. Therefore, when exercising, pay attention to hydration to prevent dryness. Drink plenty of water (preferably water with a little salt) after exercise, and drink three to four cups of water every day. Your diet should be based on the principle of nourishing *yin* and moistening the lungs, preventing dryness and protecting your *yin* energy. In addition, it is advisable for the middle-aged and elderly to take a warm bath once or twice a week in autumn, each time no more than half an hour, with the water temperature at about 25 ℃. Use soap or shower gel that does not irritate the skin. Ordinarily, it's important to also smile as much as you can. This helps not only maintain your lung *qi*, but also lifts your mood, and has been shown to help eliminate fatigue, relieve chest tightness, and restore your physical strength.

Avoid eating immediately after exercise: Fall mornings are very cold, and this can temporarily cool the nasal cavity, trachea and esophagus as the body acclimatizes to the cold. If you eat hot food for breakfast, such as porridge or hot coffee, immediately after exercise, the capillaries and slightly larger blood vessels in the esophageal mucosa and nearby tissues can struggle to deal with the stimulation. This can cause temporary regulatory dysfunction. Therefore, after morning exercise, do not eat hot food immediately. Drink some warm water first, so that the throat and stomach have time to adapt.

Jogging

As a form of fall exercise, running doesn't have to be a race! It's a better idea to slow things down. Why? Because jogging can enhance blood circulation, improve heart function, improve blood supply to the brain and oxygen supply to the brain cells, reduce cerebral arteriosclerosis, and enable the brain to function properly. Jogging can also boost metabolism, increases your energy consumption, and can help you to lose weight and keep fit. For the elderly, jogging can greatly reduce muscle atrophy and weight gain caused by inactivity. It helps reduce the age-related degeneration of heart and lung function, as well as reducing cholesterol and arteriosclerosis, and overall prolonging life. In recent years, scientists have also found that joggers are less likely to get cancer.

Of course, outdoor jogging is actually experiencing an "air bath." If people are constantly jogging in polluted air, they can feel unmotivated and weak, and their work efficiency can decline. Therefore, both healthy and sick people should go to clean outdoor areas for exercise and aim to breathe more fresh air. It is a good time to get outside and exercise in nature. Going out in the fresh air for just one to two hours a day, taking 40 minutes to jog, will not only reduce the incidence of diseases, but also helps strengthen the physique and your overall energy.

The "[s]" Breathing Method

Many people suffer from lung problems in autumn. According

to traditional Chinese medicine, the lungs are the organ most associated with the fall. At this time of year, lung *qi* is at its most vigorous, making them more prone to disease. In autumn, therefore, we should make sure we look after our lungs. There are several simple and easy breathing exercises you can do to help encourage healthy lung function. One popular method in China is the "[s]" method. It is easy to do during any short break during your day.

The method goes like this: First, keep your head and neck straight and your eyes open and focused. Put your tongue on your upper palate, sink your shoulders and elbows, and pull your chest back. Relax your waist and crotch. Bend your knees slightly and keep your feet apart, and let your whole body relax. Calm your mind, and let everything be as it is. Force nothing. When you pronounce "[s]", the shape of your mouth naturally falls so that your lips are slightly retracted, and your upper and lower teeth do not quite touch. The tip of the tongue is inserted into the upper and lower teeth, slightly protruding. As you say "[s]", lift your hands from the front of your lower abdomen, gradually turn your palms upward until they are flat on your chest, then turn your arms outward. Point the tips of your thumbs to your throat, and then extend your left and right arms and chest to push your palms out like a bird extending its wings. Exhale out, and your arms will fall naturally and hang down at your sides. Repeat six times to regulate your breath.

Doing this can help relieve coughs, pharyngitis, rhinitis and other problems of the Taiyin Lung Meridian of Hand (LU). In the morning, you can go to a park, where you'll find plenty of fresh air and lush trees. While doing so, work to stop the seven emotions from affecting you.

Four Steps to Nourish the Lungs

Below are some ways to recuperate lung *qi* and prevent colds, coughs, asthma and other diseases. The best time to practice is around 10 am. Beforehand, open a window for half an hour to let fresh air into the room. The specific exercise steps are as follows:

① Depending on your physical condition, choose a sitting or standing position. Relax your body, close your eyes slightly, and breathe evenly. Then, use an abdominal breathing method to inhale slowly through the nose. When the inhalation reaches its maximum, exhale slowly through the nose, grit your teeth gently, and say "ah" gently. Your voice should be clear and natural. After all the breath is exhaled, inhale through the nose. Repeat this 24 to 32 times in a row. This method has the effect of tonifying the lung and replenishing *qi*.

② Maintain the same posture. Keep your upper body straight, lift your chin up and lean your head back, stretching your neck, thumb and other four fingers apart. Then, use the part between your thumb and your index finger to massage your throat all the way down to your chest. Rub with the left and the right hand alternately, 40 to 60 times. This method has the effect of clearing the throat, relieving coughs and getting rid of phlegm.

③ Sit on a bed or chair. Straighten your waist and back, relax your whole body, and breathe evenly. Then, naturally cross your legs and raise them off the ground. Bend over, lowering your head forward, and put your hands on either side of your body on the bed or chair. Support your body on your arms, and arch your shoulder and back up as much as possible. Repeat five to ten times according to your physical strength. This method helps circulate lung *qi* and regulates water passages, effectively helping regulate the function of lung *qi*.

④ Take a sitting position. Relax the waist and back naturally, close your eyes and ball your hands into empty fists. Stretch your hands over to the back and hit your back, first in the center of the back, then at both sides. Move from top to bottom, then from bottom to top. Repeat three to five times. Do not hold your breath while performing this massage-like hitting. Next, click your teeth five to ten times and then slowly swallow the saliva that builds up. This method can relax the *qi* in your chest, helping unblock the back meridians, and helping nourish the lungs and stomach.

Abdominal Breathing

The lungs are the gateway by which *qi* enters the human body. They are our "first guard." The function of the lungs is mainly respiratory. They work 24 hours a day, day and night, and need to breathe evenly and smoothly. If lung function decreases for any reason, this is referred to as "lung *qi* deficiency" in traditional Chinese medicine. Lung deficiencies not only affect the generation of *qi* in the body and breathing, but also causes the symptoms of general *qi* deficiency such as a weak voice, general fatigue and physical weakness. Once the lung loses its respiratory function, clear air cannot be inhaled and toxins cannot be exhaled. *Qi* cannot be generated, which is a life-threatening situation. Therefore, it is vital to take care of our lungs and make sure we are always breathing healthily!

Abdominal breathing is a good way to encourage lung health. The specific method for doing this is: Close your mouth, gently clench your teeth together, and breathe deeply into the *dan tian* region, or elixir field in your abdomen. Hold for a few seconds, and slowly exhale. Breathing through the nose helps filter out various foreign substances. The elixir field is 3 cun below your navel. *Qi* sinks into the elixir field, and the abdomen bulges when you inhale deeply with your abdominal muscles. With the practice of this breathing technique, slowly your lungs will get into the habit of abdominal breathing, creating a strong respiratory system.

3. Leisure in Fall

Leisure time plays an important role in traditional Chinese healthy living. In the coolness of fall, what recreational activities are best to help you relax physically and mentally? How can we harmonize the flows of *qi* and blood in our body, and keep physically fit?

Tai Chi

It is a common sight in China to see people practicing Tai Chi in parks, squares, woods, gardens and other quiet outdoor places with nice scenery, open space and fresh air. When practicing Tai Chi, you should follow a step-by-step approach according to your own physique. When you're just starting out, try practicing specific movements, and gradually complete a set. If you are unwell, you should rest as much as you need to. It is not a good idea to practice when you have just eaten, or after you have consumed alcohol.

The basic principle of Tai Chi practice is as follows: First, you must stand upright. Second, you must calm your mind. Your mind should guide your movement. You must also breathe *qi* into your elixir field. Movements should be slow and deliberate, and done at an even speed. The aim of Tai Chi is to combine your inner world (your spirit) with the outside world (physical form). Movements should always match upward and downward motion; be coherent and lively; and you must breathe naturally as you practice.

Reading

There are many advantages of reading. Most people only see it as a way of expanding your knowledge and furthering your career, while ignoring its function as entertainment, or a way to help regulate your mood and improve your health.

Reading has a great influence on people's spirit and physical health. A good book draws the reader into its world, allowing them to go on a journey that can be wildly exciting and engaging.

The essence of human aging is cell aging, especially brain cell aging. A healthy brain grows stronger when it is used often, and degenerates when it is not used. Reading is exercise for your brain, and helps improve brain function and your conscious mental activity. A strong brain leads to a long life. Reading not only enriches your knowledge, but also cultivates your personality. It's a double benefit, allowing you to both maintain your health and prolong your life.

Dancing

Dance is not just a form of entertainment, it's also a great way
to exercise. It's a form of creative expression, and a workout
that benefits your health. Through movement of the body,
emotion can be expressed in action. As well as being enjoyable
as an experience, dancing also moves your joints, circulates *qi*
and blood, nourishes the blood vessels, and achieves the effect
of lightening the body, restoring physical and mental strength.
It can even improve your digestive function, help cure diseases
and prolong your life. The muscular system, nervous system,
respiratory system and cardiovascular system are all stimulated
by dance movements.

Since ancient times, Chinese people have learned to use
dance to keep fit and cure diseases. Generations of doctors and
health practitioners have constantly supported the use of dance
therapy, accumulating a large amount of treatment experience
that we still use today. First of all, dancing itself is a fantastic
form of full-body physical exercise. Studies show that the energy
consumption of even slow dancing in a social dance group is
three to four times higher than that of people in a resting state.
Secondly, when dancing, the dancer must be in time with
the music, and must concentrate mentally on the music and
dance steps. Along with the pleasurable experience of lighting
and music, dancing is an all-round highly enjoyable activity.
However, the elderly should ensure they take it easy, not trying
to do anything too complicated or fast-paced. It's also important
not to overdo it with session length.

4. What to Eat in Fall

Fall is the time to replenish the body and nourish the spirit,
making sure we have enough energy reserves for winter. China
has a common folk belief that fall is a time for "supplementing."
The word supplements often makes people think of expensive
health foods and medicines, to be added mindlessly to the diet.

Doing this, however, is extremely unscientific. It is not only useless, but may even cause you health problems, if done in the wrong way. A good way to think of diet supplementation is: spring is for birth; summer is for growth; fall is for harvesting; and winter is for storage. An important general principle is to remember that we nourish "*yang* in spring and summer, *yin* in autumn and winter." Traditional Chinese medicine views supplementing the diet as generally a good idea, but it must be done in the correct way.

Foods to Avoid

Fall is not only the best time to restore and regulate the functions of various organs of the human body, but also the best time to prepare for the coming winter.

In fall, your top priorities are looking after the spleen and stomach. In the long, hot days of summer, people often eat cold foods, which weakens the function of the spleen and stomach. If you take a large amount of diet supplements to fix this too quickly, it is a sudden increase in burden for the spleen and stomach, and this can lead to digestive organ dysfunction, chest tightness, abdominal distension, loss of appetite, diarrhea and other problems. Therefore, it is necessary to give the spleen and stomach a period of adjustment and adaptation before diving into eating rich fall foods. First, you should eat foods that are both nutritious and easy to digest that help regulate the functions of the spleen and stomach. These foods include fish, poultry eggs, yams, lotus seeds, coix seeds, etc. In addition, dairy products, beans, fresh vegetables and fruits should be eaten in an appropriate amount. Gorgon fruit is an excellent herbal supplement for this. It contains plenty of carbohydrates, proteins and other useful nutrients, and has the functions of invigorating the spleen and stomach and replenishing *qi*, building appetite, strengthening the kidneys and nourishing one's essence.

Fall weather tends to be airy, refreshingly cool, and dry. Dry air, however, can easily damage the lungs and the body's clear fluid. Therefore, one thing that a fall diet should also do is bring moisture back to the lungs. This means the foods you eat should be light-tasted. Avoid fried food, and eat many fresh vegetables and fruits. Good vegetables to eat include cabbage, spinach and cucumber; protein sources should be foods like duck and herring. It's also advisable to eat plenty of sour foods, such as sweet orange, and hawthorn berries. Always ensure you are drinking enough water. Eat plenty of radish, lotus root, bananas, pears, honey and other foods that have plenty of water in them, to help moisten the lungs and promote your body's fluid production. This helps you nourish *yin* and clear out the dryness from your body.

Your fall diet choices should also take the nature of foods into account. It is advisable to eat more warm-natured foods, and fewer cool- and cold-natured foods. This helps to protect stomach *qi*. If you eat too many cool- and cold-natured foods, such as raw or unwashed vegetables and fruit, this can lead to an accumulation of internal heat and toxins in the body. This can cause diarrhea and other stomach issues, especially in the elderly, children and the infirm.

Avoid hot, spicy and dry foods. Hot flavors mean foods such as garlic, scallion, ginger, Sichuan pepper and other spicy foods or condiments. These flavors damage your internal *yin*. This can aggravate internal heat and allow dryness pathogens to invade the body.

Avoid fried food. Fried chicken and other types of greasy foods are difficult to digest, especially in the fall. They can easily sit for a long time in your stomach, which is not good for your health. In addition, fried foods aggravate the heat accumulated in the body, which is not conducive to the body's adaptation to the characteristics of fall.

Avoid eating aquatic plants raw. Fall is the harvest season for most aquatic plants, and also high season for metacercaria that grow on them. Aquatic plants are plant foods that grow in the water, such as water caltrop, water bamboo, water chestnut and so on. Most of them are white, crisp, cool and refreshing. They taste delicious, and have the effects of clearing heat and removing toxicity. They can also improve appetite, aid digestion, help reduce phlegm and relieve coughs. However, eating these kinds of aquatic plants raw can lead to infection by Fasciolopsis buski, causing inflammation, bleeding, edema, and even ulceration of the intestinal mucosa, often accompanied by diarrhea and loss of appetite. If infected, children can develop facial edema, and their growth and mental development can even be stunted. In severe cases, infection can be fatal due to collapse or dehydration. Therefore, aquatic plants should not be eaten raw.

Salt and Honey

In autumn, the climate is dry, so the air is short of water. In the same way, the human body is also short of water, so we need to supplement this by hydrating ourselves more. Drinking plain water however is not enough to overcome this seasonal dehydration. Ancient Chinese health practitioners dealt with this seasonal problem by drinking lightly salted, boiled water during the day, and honey water in the evening. This is not only a good way to rehydrate the human body, but also a good way to maintain good overall health in fall. This simple prescription can also prevent constipation caused by autumn dryness.

Key Ingredients to Use in Fall

Duck meat: Ducks are waterfowl, and their meat is cold-natured. Nutritionists believe that once ducklings are raised to adult ducks in fall, the meat is delicious and richly nutritious. Duck meat is a very good source of protein, vitamins, calcium, phosphorus, iron and other trace nutrients essential for the human body, making it a perfect food for fall.

Lily bulbs: Lily bulbs are not only delicious, but also nutritious. They are rich in protein, vitamins, calcium, phosphorus, iron and other trace elements. Lily bulb is a highly nutritious ingredient for people of all ages. Of course, the medicinal value of lily bulbs is also very high. According to the *Compendium of Materia Medica*, lily bulbs can moisten the lungs, relieve coughs, calm the spirit, and invigorate and replenish stomach and spleen *qi*. To cook with it, ensure you clean the lily bulbs to remove any impurities, then put them in a pot, and boil in water until extremely soft. Add an appropriate amount of sugar. Wait until the soup is warm, add honey, mix it well, consuming lily bulbs in this way is very effective for lung heat and coughs.

Chrysanthemum: Chrysanthemum has a lovely fragrance, and can also be cooked in a variety of dishes. It can also be used to make tea. Chrysanthemum tea is a popular refreshing beverage. Hangzhou white chrysanthemum is particularly famous in China. It comes in two colors: yellow and white. Both are used in drinking water or tea. The flower not only has a strong and delicious aroma that can invigorate the spirit, but also has the functions of dispersing wind and clearing heat, nourishing the liver and eyes, and reducing blood pressure.

Seasonal fruits: Fall is the fruit harvest season. Pears and sugarcane in particular are very healthy to consume in this season, as they help deal with dryness. Traditional Chinese medicine believes that pears help the body produce saliva, and also quench thirst. This helps relieve coughs and excessive phlegm. They also work to clear internal heat and fire, nourish the blood, promote granulation, and hydrate the lungs and overall body. Sugarcane has the function of nourishing the body and clearing internal heat, and it is also rich in nutrients. When you're hungry after a hard day's work, eating two pieces of sugarcane is a great way to replenish your spirit. It should be noted here that since pears and sugarcane are cool in nature, people with deficiency-cold in spleen and stomach, indigestion, and postpartum blood deficiencies should not eat them. Apples, oranges, bananas, and hawthorn berries are also good to eat at this time of year.

Medicinal Food Recipes
① Congee with Chinese Yam

Ingredients: 300 g fresh yam, ten lotus seeds, three red dates, 3 g wolfberry seeds, 50 g black glutinous rice, 50 g white glutinous rice, 100 g longan pulp, one tablespoon rice wine, a small amount of rock sugar

Method: Wash the black and white glutinous rice, then soak for three to four hours. Wash the lotus seeds and put them in a bowl to soak. Wash the red dates, then soak them to soften and pit them. Wash and peel the yam, and cut it into small pieces. Pour one liter of water into a pot to boil, and add all the ingredients (except rice wine and rock sugar). Boil at high heat for ten minutes, and low heat for two hours. Add the rock sugar and rice wine, then boil until the rock sugar dissolves. Take off the heat and consume while warm.

Effects: This congee replenishes *qi* and improves blood flow, and is good for your skin, kidneys and stomach. It helps restore the function of the gastrointestinal tract.

② Glutinous Rice and Pear Congee

Ingredients: 150 g glutinous rice, half a pear, a small amount of pear peel, pear core and rock sugar

Method: First, clean the glutinous rice, keeping the rice water for use later. Put the washed glutinous rice in a bowl of clear water to soak. Soak the pear in the rice water, and wash the rind carefully with a brush. Cut the pear flesh into pieces, and set aside the core and skin on a plate. Fill a soup pot with water and heat it. Once the water is boiling, add the pear core and the soaked glutinous rice. Boil for three minutes, while stirring continuously with a spoon, and then turn to low heat to simmer. After about 15 minutes, add the pear pieces and peel, and rock sugar to taste. Bring to the boil again, then continue to simmer at low heat. Do this for about half an hour, or until the glutinous rice is soft and emits a pear fragrance. Then, turn off the heat and simmer for a moment. Pick out the pear core, and then serve.

Effects: It invigorates the spleen and stomach and replenishes *qi*, contributing to good overall health.

③ Gingko and Lily Congee

Ingredients: 50 g japonica rice, six large dates (or ten small dates), 15 g shelled walnuts, 5 g tremella, ten ginkgo fruit, ten peanuts, ten lotus seeds, 10 g lily bulbs, one pear (about 100 g), 10 g wolfberry seeds, 25 g rock sugar

Method: Wash the japonica rice, dates, peanuts, lotus seeds, lily bulbs and walnuts. Soften and wash clean the tremella with warm water. Remove the shell and skin of the ginkgo fruit, peel and core the pears, and cut both into small pieces. Place all ingredients except for the wolfberries and sugar into a soup pot and add one liter of water. Bring to the boils, then turn to low heat for 40 minutes. Wash the wolfberry seeds, then mix them in along with the rock sugar. Cook for a further 20 minutes, then serve.

Effects: It invigorates the spleen and stomach and replenishes *qi*, moistens the lungs and throat, regulates nutrient *qi* and defensive *qi*, promotes fluid production, and strengthens the kidneys and waist.

④ Cogongrass Rhizome and Honeysuckle Tea

Ingredients: 15 g honeysuckle, 25 g dried cogongrass rhizome

Method: Add one liter of water to the above ingredients, bring to a boil, and add rock sugar to taste.

Effects: It helps clear heat and remove toxicity, as well as dredging the throat. This soup is useful for viral colds, acute and chronic tonsillitis and periodontitis.

⑤ Tremella Tea

Ingredients: 20 g tremella, 5 g tea, 20 g rock sugar

Method: First wash the tremella, add water and rock sugar to stew. Soak the tea for five minutes, then take the resulting liquid and add it into tremella soup. Stir well and serve.

Effects: It nourishes *yin* and reduces internal fire, moistens the lungs and relieves coughs, particularly for coughs caused by *yin* deficiency.

5. Fall Lifestyle

The sometimes bleak weather in fall can cause some people to feel a little down. How might we adjust our lifestyle to cope with it? Traditional Chinese medicine believes that spring and summer are *yang* seasons, while autumn and winter are *yin* seasons. In the fall, we should treat the maintenance of *yin qi* in our body as a priority. We must adapt to the weather characteristics of autumn, and reduce the impact that the seasonal changes have on the *qi* in our body.

Early to Bed and Early to Rise

In fall, it's important to regulate your sleeping patterns, rising early and sleeping early. The elderly especially would do well to bed before 9 pm and get up before 6 am. Going to bed earlier helps your body draw together more *yang qi* and collect more *yin* essence. Waking up earlier helps stretch out lung *qi* and prevent excessive shrinkage of *yang qi*. At the same time, do not overwork yourself, and avoid sweating too much in daily activities. This helps prevent damage to your internal *yang qi* and *yin* fluid.

Fall nights are cool in temperature. In order to protect your body's *yang qi*, doors and windows should be kept closed as you sleep, and your midsection should always be covered with at least a thin blanket in order to prevent the spleen and stomach from getting cold. In early fall, the weather is very changeable and it's easy to catch colds. Always make sure you are wearing enough layers.

Adapting to the Cold

The Chinese medicine believes that you should not rush to take off layers in spring, nor rush to put them back on in fall. Give your body a little more time to adapt to cold in spring and feel the cold a little in fall. This is in line with the principle of "keeping warm with thin clothes" in fall, as mentioned in *The Yellow Emperor's Classic of Medicine*. However, to have a correct understanding of "adapting to the cold" in fall, we should take a step-by-step approach. This way, we strengthen the body's natural cold resistance exercise, and enhance the body's ability to adapt to natural climate changes. This helps prevent respiratory infectious diseases. In late fall, if the weather suddenly changes and the temperature drops significantly, pay attention to the weather change and make sure you're keeping warm. Adapting to the cold is beneficial, allowing the body to build an ability to resist the cold. So, feeling the chill a little in fall is a good way to be in harmony with nature.

However, deliberately exposing oneself to the cold of autumn is not suitable for the following groups of people:

Patients with cardiovascular diseases: In order to resist hypothermia, the human body must transport blood from the subcutaneous blood vessels to the body, which will lead to vasoconstriction, increased blood pressure, and accelerated cardiac pulsation. This increases the burden on the heart, increasing cardiac ischemia and hypoxia. In vulnerable individuals, this can cause coronary artery spasms and blood clots, and lead to angina pectoris or myocardial infarction.

Ulcer patients: When the human body is stimulated by the cold, histamine levels in the blood increase, as does gastric acid secretion. This can result in gastric spasm, gastric ulcer flare-ups, gastric bleeding and perforation.

Patients with cerebral blood diseases: Exposure to the cold agitates the human nervous system, causing the whole body's capillaries to contract. This increases peripheral resistance and blood pressure, conditions which can cause cerebral hemorrhage or thrombosis.

Patients with chronic lung disease: The cold air in autumn can cause adverse irritation to the respiratory tract, causing allergic reactions, induced spasm of the trachea, bronchus or bronchioles, and possible recurrence or aggravation of chronic bronchitis, bronchial asthma, and other diseases.

Arthritis patients: Wind, cold and dampness are the main things to lead to joint problems. Coldness leads to stagnation which impedes *qi* and blood flow, and these blockages lead to pain. Therefore, arthritic patients should always make sure they are keeping their legs warm from the beginning of fall, and not attempting to adapt to the cold.

Skincare

In the early autumn, the weather can still be both hot and humid. People often sweat heavily, so keeping skin clean is particularly important for skin care. However, the elderly should take care not to bath or shower too frequently, as it can dry out the skin. It is also important to not use alkaline soap. Skin pores are not only a guarding barrier of the lung, but also act as the outer surface of lung *qi*. The first place that autumn dryness can be seen is in damage to the hair follicles on the skin, making them coarse and unsightly. Make sure you are consuming plenty of healthy soups with medicinal ingredients to keep your skin hydrated and clean. Moisturizer is also beneficial.

Insulating Your Shoulders, Abdomen and Feet

The best way not to get sick when the weather turns cold is to wrap up warm. There are three key body parts that should be insulated.

Shoulders: It's very easy to injure the shoulder joint at this time of year. Anyone who has suffered from a shoulder injury in the past should be vigilant.

Abdomen: The abdomen is prone to gastrointestinal discomfort in the cool weather, resulting in abdominal pain and diarrhea. The cool getting into the abdomen is very harmful to women in particular, and can upset the menstrual cycle. It is very important therefore to always keep your midsection warm.

Feet: When the feet get cold, the whole body's resistance to the cold also decreases. In addition, the foot is also a highly sensitive and reactive part of the body. Chilly feet will cause capillary contraction in every part of the body that the foot is linked to. For people suffering from cardiovascular disease, it is particularly important to keep their feet warm.

6. Emotional Health in Fall

In autumn, there is less sunlight, the temperature is gradually falling, the grass withers and leaves fall, and flowers and trees turn dark. Many people are affected by this, as the human biological clock takes time to adapt to these rapid changes. This can lead to physiological rhythm disruptions and even endocrine disorders, and makes many people prone to sadness, depression, and other negative emotional states. Being sad is a very fast way to harm your body's *qi*. Chinese medicine phrases it this way: "Sadness dissipates *qi*." Over time, people who are in a sad emotional state will experience lower levels of immunity, and become more prone to depression. Therefore, we must pay attention to emotional health in autumn. The core of emotional health care in autumn is to do things that calm our spirit, and keep our mood in line with the "harvesting" of autumn.

Increasing Outdoor Activities

Proper exercise is highly conducive to lifting the spirit and regulating mood. When you are feeling low, go out into nature and breathe some fresh air. This helps strengthen the respiratory function and blood circulation, and has very soothing effect on the nervous system, as well as helping to eliminate boredom. Hiking for example is a good outdoor activity for the fall, and is very helpful for regulating your emotional state. Choose a fine fall day to go hiking with friends or family. Enjoy the beautiful scenery, and you will find you feel relaxed and happy, and less likely to suffer from the problems of seasonal depression.

Eating Your Way to Happiness

What you eat also has a huge effect on how you feel. In the fall, it is a great idea to eat more licorice root, red dates, lotus root, lotus seeds, wheat, longan and so on, as these foods help to nourish the mind and calm the spirit, as well as have a positive impact on feelings of anxiety and depression. Bananas are also a very good food to eat more of at this time. They are rich in potassium, magnesium and iron, vitamins which are linked to calmness and happiness. They are very helpful for improving mood.

Having Good Intentions

Having a kind heart is one of life's most important principles. Good intentions are also an indispensable method for regulating mood. Consistently kind-hearted people almost always are the way they are because they maintain a calm psychological state. This means their blood flow is in an optimal state, and they can avoid the occurrence of negative emotions such as tension, anxiety, and pessimism.

7. Physiotherapy and Health in Fall

Due to the unique climate characteristics of autumn, physical aches and pains are common in this season. These discomforts may not be enough to make you go to the hospital, but it still affects your quality of life. Here are some ways to do home massages, which are a simple, economical and practical way to improve your physical condition.

Lung Care Acupoints

Quchi acupoint: The Quchi acupoint is on the outside of the transverse lines of the elbows on both sides, and it feels sore when pressed. This acupoint is commonly used to treat exogenous diseases and has a good effect on clearing heat and purging fire. At the peak of *yang* every day (1 to 3 o'clock in the afternoon), press and knead the Quchi acupoints on both sides for two minutes. The most important thing is to do it every day. Important note: This acupoint is linked to miscarriage and should never be used on pregnant women.

Yingxiang acupoint: The Yingxiang acupoints are about 0.5 cun away from the midpoint of the outer edge of the nose, in the nasolabial groove. This point can treat various refractory rhinitis. In addition, it also has the function of moistening the nasal cavity. When the two nasal cavities are moist, this can increase resistance to pathogenic diseases, especially in the autumn when pathogenic dryness is rampant.

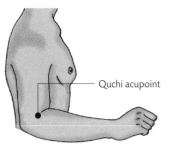

Quchi acupoint

Hegu acupoint: The Hegu acupoint is at the midpoint of the radial side of the second metacarpal bone on both hands. The simple way to select the point is to close the thumb and forefinger to find the highest point of the muscle. This acupoint is the *yuan*-primary point for the Yangming Large Intestine Meridian of the Hand (LI). Pressing and kneading this acupoint can stimulate the original *qi* of the large intestine meridian. When it is sufficient, the diseased *qi* will be eliminated.

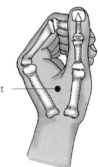

Yingxiang acupoints

Hegu acupoint

The Hegu acupoint is also linked to physical beauty. Pressure and pollution from both internal and external environments can accumulate in the body, and when these toxins begin to transform into free radicals, they can seriously affect the body, and detoxification becomes an urgent task. The deposition of toxins in the body will disrupt normal physiological functions and affect metabolism. Frequent massage of the Hegu acupoint can alleviate or eliminate the diseases of tissues and organs at the large intestine meridians, and achieve the purpose of discharging toxins accumulated in the body. The most important thing is that pressing the Hegu acupoint is

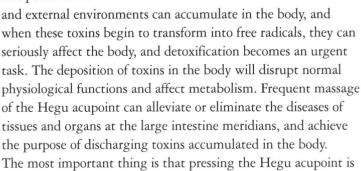

simple and easy, and you can massage it at any time, whether in a meeting or traveling in a car.

If you have a slight cold, you can also press and massage the Hegu acupoints on the left and right hands for ten minutes respectively. After, drinking a cup of hot water and sweating a little can help further relieve your cold. People with nose allergies should often massage the Hegu acupoint. Consistency in this practice can yield amazing results. In addition, because the Yangming Large Intestine Meridian of the Hand (LI) passes through the lower gums, the Hegu acupoint can also be used to relieve toothache. Important: Pressing Hegu acupoint can lead to miscarriage and should not be used for pregnant women.

Acupoints for Relieving Fatigue

Many people get sleepy in autumn and feel listless all day. According to traditional Chinese medicine, there are three health-preserving acupoints in the body, which can relieve fatigue and refresh the spirit.

Baihui acupoint: The Baihui acupoint is at the intersection of the midline of the head and the line between the two ear tips. Massaging this acupoint can refresh the spirit and increase *yang* energy. Method: Use both thumbs or forefingers to press on the Baihui acupoint, slowly and forcefully, until it feels slightly sore. Hold for 30 seconds, and at the same time, gently massage in a circular motion. Repeat five times.

Taiyang acupoint: The Taiyang acupoint is on your temples, in front of the ear, on both sides of the forehead, and above the extension line of the outer corner of the eye. Massaging this point can not only refresh your spirit, but also relieve headaches. Method: Place the thumb or forefinger of both hands on the temples on both sides, gently rotating in a circle for 30 seconds.

Fengchi acupoint: This acupoint is found at the depression between the sternocleidomastoid muscle and the upper end of the trapezius muscle, under the occipital bone of the neck on both sides. Massaging this acupoint can not only refresh you, but also relieve eye fatigue. Method: Keep your body upright, put your thumbs at the Fengchi acupoints on both sides, tilt your head back, rotate your thumbs in a circle and knead the acupoints for one minute, until you feel sore. Repeat five times.

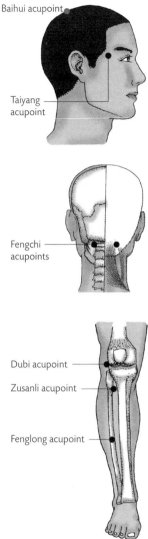

Baihui acupoint

Taiyang acupoint

Fengchi acupoints

Dubi acupoint

Zusanli acupoint

Fenglong acupoint

Gastrointestinal Acupoints

Zusanli acupoint: This point is located at the front and outside of both calves, 3 cun below the Dubi acupoint, one finger width from the front edge of the tibia. Massaging the Zusanli point can regulate the function of the spleen and stomach, promoting appetite and aiding digestion. When massaging, press with your thumb in a circular motion until it feels sore. Press 15 times each time, two to three times a day.

Fenglong acupoint: Located at the anterolateral side of the lower legs, 8 cun above the lateral ankle tip, two finger widths from the front edge of the tibia, and between the tibia and fibula. Massaging this point can strengthen the spleen and remove dampness, promote metabolism, relieve flatulence and stop hiccups. When massaging, press with your thumb in a circular motion until it feels sore. Press 15 times each time, two to three times a day.

Zhongwan acupoint: 4 cun above the navel. Massaging this acupoint can harmonize the stomach, promote *qi* flow

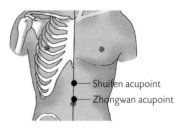

Shuifen acupoint
Zhongwan acupoint

and relieve pain, improving indigestion, stomachache and abdominal distension. When massaging, press with your thumb in a circular motion until it feels sore. Press 15 times each time, two to three times a day.

Shuifen acupoint: 1 cun above the navel. This point can promote *qi* flow and metabolism, and relieve constipation and flatulence. When massaging, press with your thumb in a circular motion until it feels sore. Press 15 times each time, two to three times a day.

Regulating Autumn Dryness

In the dry autumn season, people tend to have a low fever, dry throat, constipation and other symptoms of "excessive internal heat." If these symptoms are serious, you can utilize cupping and *gua sha* scraping treatments to clear the internal fire. First, apply some kind of lubricating oil to the body, and then carry out cupping or a scraping motion along the Taiyang Bladder Meridian of the Foot (BL) or the Jueyin Pericardium Meridian of the Hand (PC), until the skin flushes or develops red spots. This treatment should be done once a day or once every other day depending on the degree of internal fire.

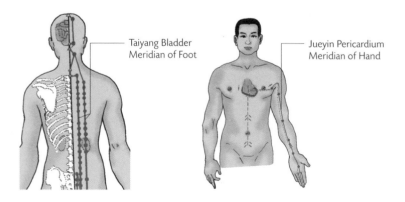

Taiyang Bladder Meridian of Foot

Jueyin Pericardium Meridian of Hand

Chapter Four
Winter

Winter is the last of the four seasons, when plants and animals begin to rest and recuperate. At this time of year, the weather becomes very cold and the vegetation withers. Nature closes in on itself, and the *yang qi* of the human body is just the same, hiding inside. Spring and summer are the time for cultivating our *yang*, while autumn and winter is the time for cultivating *yin*. Therefore, the basic principle of a healthy winter is simply to store one's energy and nourish one's *yin*.

First of all, try to go to bed slightly earlier and get up slightly later. The best time to begin your day is after the sun is already up (especially for the elderly) because, in winter, the human body needs to absorb more sunlight to supplement its *yang*. Doing too much exercise before sunrise will damage your *yang qi*. In winter, sleeping early and rising late allows you to sleep for longer, quietening your internal world and helping to keep your *yang qi* undisturbed. Another thing of great importance is making sure your back stays warm at all times. The back is the *yang* center of the human body. Wind-cold and other pathogens can easily enter the body through the back and cause diseases. The elderly, children and those of weaker health in particular should pay attention to keeping their back warm in winter to avoid damaging their body's *yang qi*. It's also of crucial and obvious importance to avoid getting too cold. When the weather is cold, everyone should be trying to stay indoors where the temperature is most comfortable, and reducing the amount of time they spend outdoors. If you do go outside, you should always make sure you are wearing warm clothes and thick shoes and socks. Keeping your feet warm is very important. Not wearing enough layers when the weather turns decreases your natural immunity, as well as the physical functional capacity of the heart, stomach, lungs and other organs. This can lead to health issues or flare-ups with existing health issues, such as tracheitis, stomachache, and even coronary heart disease. Colds, coughs, arthralgia, rheumatoid arthritis, hypertension and other diseases are also aggravated by winter weather. In addition, it should be remembered to keep warm when bathing or showering in winter. Incaution in it may cause colds and respiratory diseases. One solution to this is to reduce the number of times you bathe, and always be very mindful of the temperature of the bath water and the bathroom. Children, the elderly and anyone with existing cardiovascular or cerebrovascular diseases should be especially careful.

According to traditional Chinese medicine ideology, the lungs govern the skin and hair and the nose is the opening to all of these. If the skin is attacked by the cold, it can lead to respiratory diseases. In winter, cold weather can cause or aggravate problems with the kidneys and urinary system, leading to nephritis, enuresis, incontinence, edema and other diseases of wind chill.

From the perspective of traditional Chinese medicine, kidney is the congenital origin and "the root of five organs' *yin* and *yang*." The kidneys "store human essence," so all health-preserving attempts in winter are related to nourishing the kidney. According to the five elements theory of traditional Chinese medicine, the kidney is associated with the water element, and therefore is also associated with latent vitality and the season of storing *yang qi*. Winter is the best time to maintain and accumulate energy. Therefore, kidneys are the most important location of *yang qi* nourishment. The key to nourishing the kidney is to regulate the spirit. In order to do this, one should keep oneself relatively inward-facing, keeping oneself to oneself, so as to protect your *yang*. You should aim to not be disturbed, and to make sure that your spirit remains protected and fresh, so that the body can also be healthy in the coming year.

To sum up, traditional Chinese medicine's view of how to stay healthy in winter all lies in nourishing *yin* energy and looking after one's kidneys.

1. Prevention in Winter

Winter weather is very cold, and the human body's *yang qi* folds in on itself, similar to many other beings in nature at this time of year. Our natural immunity weakens, and the risk rises for a broad variety of problems such as respiratory disease, stomach problems, coronary heart disease, stroke, diabetes, arthritis, and internal bleeding due to cirrhosis. At this time of year, mastering some winter disease prevention knowledge is a quick way to nip these diseases in the bud.

Advice for the Elderly

In winter, the weather is cold and dry. For more vulnerable populations, especially the elderly, winter can be a testing time. Respiratory diseases, stroke and other cardiovascular and cerebrovascular diseases can become dangers.

Respiratory diseases: It is cold in winter, and the air is dry, especially when there is little snowfall. Viruses and bacteria are particularly active at this time of year. Respiratory mucosa is easily stimulated at this time of year, especially amongst the elderly, and our reduced winter immunity makes it very easy to be infected with respiratory diseases. For the elderly, colds, pneumonia and asthma are the main problems that need to be prevented in this season. Older people who smoke are advised to give up smoking during the winter, because the irritation of smoking makes them more susceptible to respiratory diseases.

Heart diseases: In winter, the elderly have relatively poor adaptability to the cold, so this period also sees a high incidence of cardiovascular diseases such as angina. Cold weather also causes blood vessels to constrict, increasing blood pressure and reducing blood supply. These conditions can cause an irregular heartbeat, angina, or even eventually lead to myocardial infarction and other serious consequences. The main manifestations of angina are chest pain and difficulty breathing. Some patients may experience toothache on one side or upper limb pain, and some female patients may also present with breathing difficulties and stomach discomfort. These symptoms may not appear serious, and patients often ignore them. Mood fluctuation is also an inducing factor for cardiovascular disease. Therefore, it is very important for the elderly to maintain a calm mind and avoid too much emotional excitement in the winter. It is not advisable to be either dramatically happy or dramatically sad.

Cerebrovascular diseases: As we age, our blood vessels become harder and less elastic. Cold, fatigue, and rapid mood swings can also cause the blood vessels to contract suddenly, resulting in insufficient blood supply, hypoxia in the brain, cerebral hemorrhage, or cerebral embolism, commonly known as "stroke." Generally speaking, strokes are divided into two types: ischemic strokes and hemorrhagic strokes, namely cerebral embolism (a blockage to blood flow to the brain) and cerebral hemorrhage (bleeding in the brain). The early symptoms of ischemic stroke include sudden dizziness, sudden half-face or body numbness, weakness, etc. Some patients also see double, and find themselves yawning frequently. Some patients' symptoms will disappear within 24 hours, and doctors call this a "minor stroke." Hemorrhagic stroke is characterized by sudden severe headaches, nausea and vomiting, amongst other symptoms.

Cold Damage to the Head

Traditional Chinese medicine believes that "the head is where all *yang* converges," and that *yang qi* is also most easily lost from the head. Just like the top of a thermos bottle, if you don't pay attention to the warmth of your head, your bodily warmth can be blown away by the wind, which can easily cause vasospasm and even facial paralysis. Sometimes, when walking around in cold winds, people get headaches. These are caused by vasoconstriction caused by the cold air. It's therefore important to keep our heads warm and protected from the cold in winter, especially for the elderly. You should always wear a suitable hat when you go outside.

Sneezing

In winter, many people find themselves sneezing after inhaling cold air. Sneezing is a normal physiological phenomenon. Rapid inhalation of cold air stimulates nasal mucus, which then produces a rapid and powerful exhalation process. This is an effective protective respiratory reflex of the human body.

Sometimes, however, a strong sneeze can actually become the cause of diseases.

① Sneezing causes a sudden increase in the pressure in the blood vessels of the head, neck and chest. For some people with latent disease risk, sneezing violently can cause blood vessels to rupture and lead to nosebleeds or internal hemorrhages.

② A sudden increase of pressure in the respiratory tract and middle ear can cause membrane ruptures.

③ Lumbar muscles injury and lumbar discs herniation can be caused by a strong sneeze-induced lumbar muscle contraction.

Seasonal Dermatosis

Skin diseases are often related to temperature and humidity, as well as what you are eating and how you are feeling your spirit. The following seasonal skin problems are particular risks in winter.

Skin pruritus: In winter, the weather is dry, meaning the skin will also be dry, easily causing pruritis. Frequent scratching can easily lead to skin inflammation, cuts, eczema, scalping off, skin thinning, and even bacterial infection, which mostly occurs in the inner thigh, the extended side of the shank, and around the joints. Pruritis is more common in the elderly and people with dry skin. It can also be brought on by bathing. If you have itchy skin, resist scratching it. Do not use hot water on it, either. Adjust the water temperature during bathing to no more than 32℃, and avoid using soaps or other detergents with strong anti-oil effects. Do not rub while bathing. Try to ensure adequate humidity in your rooms; avoid spicy and pungent foods; and use drugs to relieve itching when necessary. Additionally, try not to put yourself in high-stress or high-excitement situations. Tea leaves contain high amounts of the trace element manganese, which can protect the skin. So, for itchy skin sufferers, it is recommended to drink a little tea every day.

Winter dermatitis: In winter, the skin's pores and oil glands secrete less, coupled with dry air, skin loses moisture, and the nerve endings under the skin are also blunted. Dermatitis is therefore very common. Elderly people's sebaceous gland and skin renewal functions are reduced, so they are even more likely to experience this problem. For dermatitis, we can adjust the humidity of the indoor environment by using humidifiers and growing indoor plants. This helps alleviate the dehydrated skin condition. Don't bathe too often, and when you do wash, the water should not be too hot, otherwise, the natural protective film of sweat and oil formed on your skin by your pores will be lost, leading to your skin becoming even drier. It's also a good idea to eat less shrimp, crab, beef, mutton and other similar foods. If the dermatitis is related to congenital ichthyosis or diabetes, or accompanied by constipation or cholecystitis, seek medical attention. At the same time, remember to wear loose, comfortable underwear. Pure cotton products are the best.

Chapped hands and feet: This is another common skin disease in winter. This disease is related to heredity, but can also be seen in people whose diet lacks certain vitamins. For chapped hands and feet, the most important prevention measure is keeping the cold out. Hands and feet should be protected by layers at all times, and your clothes, shoes and socks should be loose and always dry. Chapped skin can take a long time to heal, due to the thick cuticles in the diseased area. Utilize gentle anti-cracking creams or gels. People with allergies should also try taking vitamin supplements, and reduce skin contact with any acid and alkaline chemical products.

Cold urticaria: People with cold urticaria will have itching and erythema, and wind clumps appearing all over the body after exposure to cold. Some patients only have these reactions in parts of the body that are exposed to cold (such as the face and hands). Generally, the hives reaction will occur within a few minutes after exposure to cold, and will subside naturally after 20 minutes of being warmed up again, leaving no traces. Hives can recur, however, with some sufferers finding the itching completely unbearable. To avoid hives, always try to keep exposed parts of the body (such as the face, neck and hands) warm, and wear hats and gloves. Other parts of the body should also be kept warm, avoiding direct contact with cold wind and cold water. Adjust your eating habits and try to avoid eating high-protein foods such as fish, shrimp, crab, and mutton, as well as pungent foods such as wine. It's also a good idea to do more exercise, so our bodies are stronger to adapt to the changes between hot and cold.

Eczema: Eczema is an inflammatory reaction on the skin, caused by parasympathetic nerve stimulation that affects immune function in the body. It is a common skin disease. In the cold and dry winter period, many people use more moisturizer and external skin care products, and often eat spicy foods to help stave off the cold. As a result, many patients suffer from eczema. To prevent this, avoid taking hot water baths or using alkaline body wash. Do not scratch affected areas, and focus on eating less spicy and pungent foods. You should also try hard to keep the skin clean.

Exfoliative keratolysis: Exfoliative keratolysis is also a common skin disease in winter. Sufferers will notice flaky, peeling skin on their hands and feet in winter. In severe cases, keratolysis can be painful and skin can flush. Symptoms can be treated by supplementing compound vitamin B or applying urea ointment externally.

Chapped Lips

Winter weather is cold and dry, and many people get dry lips. How can they be treated and prevented?

It's all about drinking enough water. In dry weather, your body is prone to dehydration, both internally and externally. Taking in a sufficient amount of water is always helpful to the function of the human body, and this simple step can effectively prevent the occurrence of dry lips.

Eat more fresh fruits and vegetables. For example, vegetables such as soybean sprouts, oilseed rape, Chinese cabbage, and white radish can act as vitamin B supplements; sugarcane, banana, watermelon, pear, apple and other fruits can effectively nourish *yin* and promote fluid production, as well as supplement vitamins A and B. These are effective cures for chapped lips.

Correct bad habits such as licking and biting lips. Licking your lips with your tongue will only accelerate the occurrence of dry cracks.

Wear a mask for prevention. Wearing a mask can maintain a stable temperature and humidity in your lip area, and can also help you avoid any influence from the external environment such as wind and sun damage.

Use lip balms or oils. Balms, oils, honey, chilblain cream, or colorless lipstick can all be used to help protect your lips. For people with a lot of allergies, applying balm or honey to their lips with cotton swabs can also have a good moisturizing effect.

If chapped and scabbed lips do not heal, seek medical attention.

2. Exercise for Winter

Many people are less willing to exercise in winter, when it's very cold outside. But as an old Chinese saying about winter goes: "More movement means less illness; less movement means more medicine." This is a demonstration of the common knowledge that physical exercise in winter is very beneficial to health.

Precautions for Winter Exercise

There are some things to remember, however, since improper exercise in winter can actually cause rather than prevent disease.

① In winter, the best form of exercise is mainly indoor, but it is also advisable to walk outside occasionally to get some fresh air into the lungs. Being outside also exposes your body to some of the natural winter cold, which in small doses is beneficial and harmless.

② When exercising outdoors, however, always wait for the sun to be out. The three deep winter months are a "closed off" season. This means that *yang qi* is closely guarded inside the body, while *yin* energy is on the outside. That's why we sleep for longer periods during the winter. The same logic applies to not going out if the sun is not shining.

③ Don't overdo anything during winter exercise. Doing physical exercise in winter is very beneficial to health. However, if we do not pay attention to hygiene while working out, it can actually cause harm. It is easy to catch a cold in winter. If you have a cold or fever, do not engage in strenuous exercise. Otherwise, it will aggravate the disease and can even induce myocardial infarction or myocarditis.

④ Don't forget to warm up before exercise. In cold conditions, the muscles of the human body are stiff and the flexibility of joints is poor. If you don't warm up before exercise, it's all too easy to strain a muscle or joint.

Power Walking

Fast-paced walking is a great form of exercise in winter. The weather is perfect for it, since when it's cold outside, we involuntarily accelerate our pace when walking outside anyway. However, there is a right and a wrong way to do this. When power walking, you should always try not to hunch, instead, raising your head high and keeping your chest out. Try to swing your arms wide, and keep your paces long.

When people are walking, their muscular systems

function like a pump, pushing blood through the heart. Power walking can speed up your muscular reactions, promoting blood circulation throughout the body and increasing oxygen consumption. It's also a workout for your heart as a muscle, which is very helpful in improving circulation problems to the extremities that are specific to winter. Frequent power walking is also an effective weight loss tool.

Spending too much time in air-conditioned rooms can give people "AC syndrome." Therefore, it's far better to warm up with exercises such as walking, which not only drive away the cold but also strengthen the body.

Rubbing the Hands Together

In the cold winter weather, frequently rubbing your hands together has two benefits:

① It can prevent frostbite. Some women and children have poor blood circulation, and are very prone to frostbite if the temperature drops below 10℃. Without exercise or effective warming measures, frostbite can easily occur in the fingers, backs of the hands, feet, ears, cheeks and so on. Frequently rubbing your hands together helps both increase local temperature by creating heat from friction, and also accelerate blood circulation, thus fundamentally preventing frostbite.

② Frequently rubbing the hands together can promote blood circulation and metabolism and prevent colds. The root of the thumb of both hands is called thenar, and is an effective area for treating respiratory diseases. Several acupoints converge at this area, and stimulating it helps promote blood circulation, dredge the body's meridians, and strengthen the natural immune ability of the face, throat, nose and upper respiratory tract.

Rubbing the Face

Rubbing the face not only helps stretch out facial nerves and muscles, but also helps prevent facial nerve inflammation (neuritis), vision loss and rhinitis, and prevent colds. The facial nerves are very numerous, but fragile, and are prone to neuritis due to the high number of external factors that the face is exposed to. Symptoms of neuritis can be a slanted mouth, lower eyelid ectropion, or even difficulty eating soup or rice. Therefore, it's very important that we look after our facial nerves. In addition to strengthening our overall physical condition and preventing wind-cold pathogens from invading the body, regularly rubbing the face is a very effective maintenance measure. Because rubbing the face can speed up blood circulation, it helps activate and nourish the facial muscles and nerves. At the same time, blood circulation around the eye will also be accelerated, which helps not only alleviate visual fatigue, but also enhances the vitality of the optic nerve, slowing down degenerative eye diseases. When rubbing the face, you can also massage your nose, helping promote blood circulation in the nasal cavity. This stops dryness, and can effectively prevent colds and rhinitis.

Foot Rubs

Rubbing the soles of your feet every day can have great benefits on the brain and kidney, helping strengthen the mind and calm the spirit. Foot rubs activate blood circulation, unblocking blood vessels, and help prevent colds, forgetfulness, insomnia, indigestion, loss of appetite, abdominal pain, constipation, and problems with the heart, liver, spleen, gall bladder and other organs. Foot rub methods include:

Dry foot rub: Hold the front of the left instep with the left hand, and rub along the soles of the foot with the right hand 100 times. Then, hold the right foot with your right hand and rub up and down the center of your foot with your left hand 100 times.

Wet foot rub: Put your feet in a warm water basin, soak them until they flush red, and then massage as described above.

Foot rub with alcohol: Pour about 25 grams of spirit into the cup, dip your hand in some of it, then use the hand to rub the feet as described above. Dip your hand in the alcohol again as soon as it dries. Rub both feet 100 times.

Tiptoe Exercise

Ancient Chinese doctors and health care practitioners had long recognized the importance of blood circulation in the lower limbs, so they invented corresponding physiotherapy methods, one of which is tiptoe exercise. Tiptoe exercises are part of *ba duan jin*, a school of *qigong* exercise.

Method: Put your feet together on the ground, lift your heels quickly, and then relax. Repeat 20 to 30 times. This is a simple but very effective method for improving physical fitness. When you stand on your tiptoes, the amount of blood squeezed out by the muscles at the back of both shanks each time they contract is roughly equal to the amount of blood output of a heartbeat. So, this is a great exercise to perform when doing something like playing chess, playing cards, sitting at your computer, or standing still for a long time. Try to do this exercise once every hour or so, to ensure good blood flow in the lower limbs. These tiptoe exercises also encourage movement in the limbs and activity in the brain, reducing dizziness or vision issues caused by standing too quickly after extended periods of concentration.

Exercises that Nourish the Kidney

(1) Place the thumb on the palm of the hand, with your thumb tip at the root of the ring finger. Bend your other four fingers, and hold the thumb firmly with a little force. Raise your heels, gripping the floor with all five toes; your legs should be together, with your buttocks raised, abs contracted and shoulders down. Bring your heels to the ground first, without bending your knees;

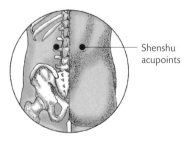

Shenshu acupoints

then, sit down on the edge of a chair or bed. Rub your palms together until they are hot, then press them on your back and waist, and massage the Shenshu acupoints on your back up and down until you feel the heat spread through you.

② Rub the palms of your hands to make them hot, then use them to rub the center of your right foot with your left hand and the center of left foot with your right hand. Every morning and evening, do this about 300 times. Regular massage of the Yongquan acupoint benefits the kidneys and the human body's essence, as well as soothing the liver and improving eyesight. It helps sleep, strengthens the body, and has anti-aging effects. In addition, massaging this acupoint can also help to treat dizziness, insomnia, tinnitus, headache and other diseases caused by kidney deficiencies.

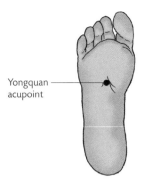

Yongquan
acupoint

③ Pinch the tips of your ears between your thumb and forefinger, and lift, pull, knead, pinch and rub 15 to 20 times until the area flushes red and becomes hot. This method is calming and can soothe pain, clear the mind, improve eyesight, and reduce internal heat. It also has anti-allergy and kidney-nourishing effects, and can prevent and treat hypertension, insomnia, pharyngitis and skin diseases.

3. Leisure in Winter

Traditional Chinese medicine believes that the arrival of winter is a time when *yin qi* is at its peak, and *yang qi* recedes along with the leaves and insects. Winter is a time for supplementing the diet and nourishing the kidneys to protect against the cold. In winter, individuals should aim to "reset" the body. Doing so not only helps pass the winter smoothly, but also helps us "conserve essence and accumulate energy." Traditional Chinese medicine has a common saying "In autumn and winter, we nourish *yin*." Especially in winter, looking after one's health means paying attention to "conservation." Spring is associated with rebirth; summer with growth; autumn with harvests and winter with storage. This is the law of nature. If we spend every winter prioritizing the "storage" of energy in our bodies, we can effectively prevent and treat many diseases, and pass the winter in a very pleasant way.

Hot Springs

Hot spring water is hot and pungent in nature, and this can promote the smooth movement of *qi* and make the body sweat and detoxify. Heat can warm and activate the meridians, unblock *qi* and blood flows, and enhance organ function. This helps balance *yin* and *yang* in the body and refreshes the spirit. Bathing in the hot springs and being exposed to their water temperature, pressure and buoyancy can improve the responsiveness of the nervous system, and also helps the expansion of peripheral blood vessels, accelerating blood circulation. This boosts metabolism, reduces muscle tension and fatigue, and can help relieve spasms and pains. There are many kinds of hot springs, and each may contain different natural minerals such as sulphion, hydrogen sulfide, sulfate, phosphorus, calcium, potassium, magnesium, fluorine, iron, boron, iodine, radon and many other elements. Each has different curative effects. For example, pure springs which contain various trace elements are not taxing on the body, and have a broad scope of recuperation effects. It can help the symptoms of neurasthenia, neuralgia, rheumatism, and skin diseases. Hot springs containing calcium, magnesium and other hydrogen carbonates have calming effects that can be helpful in combating high blood pressure, and also improve physical fitness and restore physical strength. Hot springs with high concentration of bicarbonate of soda can help moisturize and beautify the skin; while acidic hot springs containing hydrogen sulfide, green alum, carbon dioxide and other ingredients can soften the cuticles and have strong antibacterial effects. Acidic springs may also help patients with skin diseases such as scabies, ringworm, chronic eczema, acne, prurigo, scleroderma, neurodermatitis, and so on. Hot springs containing radioactive elements radon and radium have a soothing effect on the nerves, and can adjust heart rate and blood pressure to healthy levels. Such springs are an effective therapy for patients with diabetes, neuralgia, rheumatism, gout and gynecological diseases.

Indoor Yoga

Since the air is dry and cold in winter, which can be irritating to the respiratory tract, winter is not a suitable time for strenuous exercise. Instead, it's best to do some simple and comfortable exercise indoors. Yoga is a very good choice. Yoga balances the nervous system and relieves psychological pressure through postures, breathing and meditation. Its movements are very slow and won't cause much sweating. Long-term yoga practice can help regulate organ function, expel toxins from the body, and make the body flexible. It is very suitable for practice in winter and can help stretch out your tendons, too.

Bowling

Many people think of bowling as a form of entertainment, but it is also very beneficial as an exercise for the body and mind. When done right, bowling utilizes more than 200 muscles in the body. A cold and windy winter day is a great time to go bowling with a group of friends. As well as exercising, this activity can help reduce stress, while avoiding the respiratory irritation that might be caused by outdoor winter sports.

Skiing

Skiing is a quintessential winter sport. As well as being fast-paced and fun, it also helps train your balance, coordination and flexibility. Skiing does not have to be an intense activity, and involves the muscles of the whole body. Skiing is a workout for your head, neck, hands, wrists, arms, shoulders, waist, legs, knees, ankles and almost all joints of the human body. It helps reduce stiffness and enhance the flexibility of the body, as well as helping reduce excess fat.

4. What to Eat in Winter

This book has previously discussed that the key to the winter diet is "supplementation." However, many people have misconceptions about this. Many people think that supplements have to be expensive and difficult to find before they can really play a role in health. In fact, the effectiveness of supplements has very little to do with their price. Some very common foods can play a huge role in health preservation. The key is knowing what they do and how to consume them properly. A good winter diet should feature reduced amounts of salty food and increased bitter foods. This helps nourish heart *qi* and maintain intercourse between the heart and kidney. You should always avoid eating too many raw and cold foods in winter, as this can easily damage the spleen and stomach *yang qi*.

Winter Supplement Foods

Medicinal supplements are always secondary to foods. There are many kinds of foods which act as healthful medicine, and these can be roughly divided into the following three categories.

Cereals: Such as glutinous rice, soybeans, peanuts and sesame seeds. Drinking wine made from glutinous rice can nourish the blood and skin, remove dampness and promote blood circulation, and stop chills from causing stomach pain. Soybeans contain many healthy fats and micronutrients, and they also have a protein content of up to 40%. Peanuts are not only high in protein, but also contain arginine, histidine, lecithin, purine, betaine, cellulose, and vitamins A, B, E, and K, which are extremely beneficial to the human body. They also taste delicious in many different dishes. Sesame seeds contain protein, fat, calcium, phosphorus, iron and many more trace elements. They contain healthy unsaturated fatty acids, which are associated with anti-aging, and longer life for the elderly.

Meats: Good winter meats include mutton, beef, chicken, quail, pigeon, and so on. Mutton is a wonderful health food for protection against the cold. It helps "replenish *qi* and strength, protect against consumptive disease, strengthen *yang*, stimulate appetite and strengthen the kidneys." Beef helps nourish the kidney and fortify the body's *yang* energy. Eating beef helps combat impotence, low libido, and limbs that struggle to stay warm. Black-bone chicken is a very good choice at this time of year. Its meat contains 17 different kinds of amino acids, seven of which are essential for the human body, and it has many highly nutritious varieties. Black-bone chicken is especially nourishing for the elderly, weak, sick or disabled. Quail is sometimes known as the "ginseng in animal world," i.e., an all-round healer. Pigeon meat is also said to be "worth nine chickens," and is a rare and valuable health supplement in winter.

Fruits and nuts: Including walnuts, chestnuts, pine nuts, red dates, ginkgo fruit, lotus seeds, longans, etc. Walnuts have high fat content, and 70% are linoleic acid and linolenic acid, which can expel cholesterol from the body. Eating just three walnuts a day can reduce the risk of heart disease. One hundred grams of chestnuts contain 70 grams of sugar and starch, five to ten grams of protein, six grams of fat, and various vitamins and inorganic salts. These help fortify the kidney and spleen. Pine nuts, also known as "evergreen nuts," can not only prolong life, but also have beautifying and anti-aging properties, and can help make human skin and hair smoother and more hydrated.

Red dates also deserve a special mention here. Also known as jujube, red dates have a sugar content as high as 80%, and the content of vitamin C ranks first among fruits, 100 times higher than apples and peaches, and ten times higher than oranges. They are sometimes called a "natural multivitamin." Red dates are a very common traditional health food in China, known for their benefits to the spleen and stomach. Red dates help replenish *qi* and aid blood flow, as well as calm the spirit and regulate overall health. They are especially effective for those with *qi* and blood flow issues. Ginkgo fruit, lotus seeds and longans are also good for human health in winter.

Seasonal foods have always been considered best for health.

Here are some winter "specialties" that you will spot throughout the winter.

Pumpkin: Pumpkin is one of winter's most versatile vegetables, which can be steamed, roasted, fried, or boiled. Its bright orange color comes from its high level of β carotene, a powerful antioxidant that helps prevent heart disease and cancer.

Grapefruit: Sour, sweet and juicy, grapefruit is the "perfect fruit" for winter. Grapefruit is not only rich in vitamin C, but also contains lycopene, both of which are powerful antioxidants and have anti-cancer effects.

Purple cabbage: There are many varieties of cruciferous vegetables, and purple cabbage is one of the most nutritious for winter. It is not only rich in vitamins, but also famous for its amazing anti-inflammatory effects. Eating raw or boiled purple cabbage is a good way to prevent cardiovascular disease and cancer.

Broccoli: Broccoli can provide vitamins A, C, K and folic acid, as well as essential minerals such as calcium, manganese and iron. It is also rich in lutein, which helps protect the eyes and reduce the occurrence of cataract and macular degeneration.

Sweet potato: Sweet potato has an arguably better nutrition profile than standard potatoes. A medium-sized sweet potato contains about four grams of dietary fiber and about two grams of vegetable protein. Moreover, sweet potatoes are very low in calories and contain almost no fat.

Chestnut: Chestnut is a healthy dried fruit that's a delicious snack throughout winter. They are rich in B vitamins and minerals such as potassium, copper and manganese, which can strengthen the body. They are also the only nuts that contain vitamin C, and so are a very good snack when colds and flu are prevalent.

Garlic: Garlic contains allicin, which is effective in preventing diseases, especially cancer and heart disease. Garlic also has anti-inflammatory and anti-bacterial properties.

White-Colored Foods

A good rule of thumb is to eat more white-colored food in

winter. According to traditional Chinese medicine, this is one method of moistening the body, often used to relieve dryness and internal heat. According to the five elements and five colors theory, white foods are best for preventing dryness and heat in the body. When cooking, try to include ingredients such as white radish, cabbage, white gourd, lily bulbs, white fungus and lotus root. Amongst these, cabbage and white radish have the best effect, and they are also very economical. However, those suffering from stomach chills should not eat them often.

Black-Colored Foods

Traditional Chinese medicine theory links the color black to the water element, which is associated with the kidney of the human body. The kidney is the source of life, and the vital gate of the body. Black is a color that expresses youth and vitality, which is why traditional Chinese medicine views foods that are naturally black in color as a winter supplement since ancient times. The melanin contained in plants that are black has beautifying, nourishing and anti-aging effects, and helps with disease prevention, cancer prevention and overall fitness.

Healthy black-colored foods for winter: Black rice and purple glutinous rice both help nourish the blood, stimulate appetite and encourage *qi* flow. Shiitake mushrooms help nourish the stomach and spleen. Black sesame strengthens the body, replenishes internal organs and *qi*, tonifies kidney *yin* and nourishes the bone marrow. This makes it highly beneficial to the liver, kidneys and blood, helping reduce dryness, and adding shine to the hair. It is an excellent food for overall health care, disease prevention and as a beauty supplement.

Black foods that keep your body warm: Black-colored foods also help warm and replenish kidney *yang*, warming the body by producing heat, and driving out the cold. Those who feel the cold especially sharply in winter should eat more warm- and hot-natured foods all year round. These include many kinds of black-colored foods, and iron-rich foods, such as animals' organ meats like liver and kidney, black fungus, mushroom, sea cucumber, kelp and oyster. Increasing your intake of iron and iodine in this way can enhance the body's hematopoietic and thermogenic functions, which helps combat anemia and greatly enhance the oxygen-carrying capacity of the blood. This increases the vitality of the whole body and overall energy levels.

Black foods can enhance immune function: Fermented black beans contain large amounts of urokinase, which can dissolve blood clots. They, therefore, are extremely effective in preventing and treating senile dementia and hypertension. Black mushrooms and shiitake mushrooms contain a lot of polysaccharides, a variety of active enzymes, and high amounts of anti-carcinogen selenium, which can improve immunity and also effectively prevent hypertension, hyperlipidemia, coronary heart disease and diabetes.

Honey

Honey is a great supplement for skin care, beauty and digestion. The dry weather of winter can easily lead to dry skin. At this time, honey can be used to make delicious honey and milk beverages, honey and snow pear water, banana and honey porridge and so on, which all help nourish *yin* energy. Honey also helps relieve constipation. It's a great thing to eat more of in the dry winter season. Below are several ways to incorporate honey into your diet.

Honey and milk drink: 50 ml honey, 50 ml milk, 25 g black sesame. First, crush the black sesame, then mix it with honey and milk. Consume with warm boiled water on an empty stomach in the morning. This sweet and delicious drink is suitable for postpartum blood deficiencies, intestinal dryness, constipation, sallow complexion, and skin dryness.

Banana and honey congee: Take 50 to 100 g of rice, 200 g of banana, and some honey. Simmer the rice into congee on the stove, cut the banana into small pieces and add them in. After it has cooled, add the honey just before you eat it. This mixture helps hydrate the intestines and relieve constipation, as well as nourishing *yin* energy.

Honey and snow pear water: Take one to two snow pears (also known as Sydney pears) and peel and cut them into pieces. Place the pieces into a stew cup and steam in a pot with a little water for about one hour. Take the cup out to cool, add two spoons of honey and stir well. Drinking pear water and eating pear flesh helps nourish the lungs and hydrate the body. It can alleviate dry mouth, thirst, dry throat and other problems caused by winter dryness.

Honey and radish juice: Wash and peel 400 g of white radish, then cut into pieces and wrap with clean gauze to extract the juice. Take 60 ml of this juice per serving and mix with one spoonful of honey before consuming. Take three times a day for three to five days for effective constipation relief.

Honey water: Simply add two spoons of honey to warm water (below 40 °C). This can quickly replenish energy. Drinking honey water after exercise or staying up late can relieve fatigue.

Mutton

Mutton meat is warm but not dry in nature. It has the function of tonifying the kidney and strengthening *yang*, as well as warming the body and dispelling the cold. It is an important supplement food in winter. So, how should you eat mutton?

In soups, stews, or steamed: These preparation methods help ensure that nutrients are not lost, resulting in a better nourishing effect. When stewing, first cook the leg bones and vertebrae of the mutton for half an hour on high heat, until the broth is milky white. Then, remove the bones and cook the washed mutton meat in the pot. Add shallots and ginger to stew. If stewed in a casserole, the flavor is better. If you like meaty dishes, braising and steaming are good options for mutton, because it preserves the nutritional value of the meat. Those who prefer to drink soup should stew mutton, so the best nutrition goes into the liquid. Having different ways of eating supplementary foods helps you satisfy your appetite at the same time as your health.

Stir-fried mutton: This method has the effect of tonifying *qi* and deficiencies, warming the body, and sweating to detoxify. This recipe makes mutton tender and delicious, without the muttony smell. It is oily and rich, and has a lasting aftertaste. Here's how to make it:

Ingredients: 300 g sliced mutton, 30 g onion, eight spring onions, four cloves of garlic, starch to taste

Seasoning: 45 g edible oil, two teaspoons sesame oil, one tablespoon soy sauce, 1/2 tablespoon white vinegar, three teaspoons white sugar, one teaspoon monosodium glutamate

Method: Mix the mutton with the soy sauce, monosodium glutamate and starch, marinate for ten minutes, pour out the excess sauce, and drain. Wash the onions and cut into pieces. Wash and slice the garlic. Wash and cut the scallions. Add oil to the pot, heat it, then add the mutton and stir fry for one minute, then remove from the heat. Add oil to the frying pan, pour in the onions, garlic and scallions, stir fry for two minutes until fragrant, then stir fry the fried mutton together, and add the white vinegar, sesame oil and sugar. Stir-fry all the ingredients in the wok for two minutes and then spread them evenly across a flat-bottomed iron frying pan. Cook on high heat, then add the starch to thicken the sauce before serving.

Sliced mutton hot pot: Sliced mutton hot pot can not only protect against the cold, but also nourish the body. It is very suitable for eating in winter. The key to this recipe is that soaking mutton in cold water overnight helps remove the mutton smell. However, what needs to be remembered is that boiled mutton in spicy soup is a very hot-natured dish and can lead to excessive internal heat. Therefore, you could add some ingredients that reduce heat and dryness, such as tremella or pears, or drink some chrysanthemum tea, to reduce the heat. Mutton should be carefully selected and boiled thoroughly, to make sure it does not contain germs or parasites.

Radish

Radish contains large amounts of water and vitamin C, as well as a small amount of protein, and a certain amount of micronutrients such as calcium, phosphorus, iron, sugar, lignin, choline, oxidase, glycosidase, catalase, amylase, mustard oil and other beneficial ingredients. According to traditional Chinese medicine, radishes are cool in nature and pungent and sweet in taste. They enter the lung and stomach meridians, and can dissipate blockages, as well as remove phlegm and heat. Radish helps *qi* move lower in the body, helps detoxify, and can be used to relieve indigestion and abdominal distention, and combat urination problems. All of these properties are why radish is sometimes called "mini ginseng."

Carrots nourish the stomach. Carrots are called the "affordable ginseng" of the radish family. Traditional Chinese medicine believes that carotene, found in high amounts in carrots, helps nourish vital energy, and strengthen the intestines and stomach. It also strengthens original *yang*, and soothes the five internal organs. At the same time, it also contains abundant alanine, calcium, phosphorus, iron and other minerals, which have obvious effects on protecting eyesight and promoting children's growth and development. In the dryness of winter, eating carrots also has a well-known beautifying effect, hydrating the skin.

White radish moistens the lungs and stops coughing. White radish is cool-natured and refreshing, and has the effect of moistening the lungs and relieving coughs. Especially in winter, people often experience symptoms such as excessive phlegm due to internal dryness-heat, pulmonary discomfort, etc. Eating some sugared white radish is a good home remedy. In addition, when white radish is eaten raw, its pungent nature can help promote the secretion of gastric juices, regulating gastrointestinal function and producing a good anti-inflammatory effect. Modern research has found that the mustard oil and glucoside contained in white radish can interact with a variety of enzymes and are effective anti-carcinogens.

Green radish strengthens the spleen and helps with

weight loss. Green radishes contain a large amount of amylase, protein, potassium and other minerals, which have the effects of invigorating the spleen, eliminating phlegm, and promoting clear fluid production. Moreover, green radish also contains few calories and a lot of fiber, which is very filling without being fattening. This makes it a great food for weight loss. In addition, the refined fiber in green radish can promote gastrointestinal peristalsis and help to discharge the waste in the body. Regular consumption of green radish can also reduce blood lipids, soften the blood vessels, stabilize blood pressure, and prevent coronary heart disease, arteriosclerosis, cholelithiasis and other diseases.

Water radish can dissolve alcohol and aid digestion. Water radish is the fresh root of radish, a cruciferous plant. Stir-fried, boiled or eaten raw are all good. It's delicious when eaten raw as a fruit, and it can also be pickled. Water radish is rich in nutrition and has very good culinary and medicinal value. It is a natural diuretic, and so is good for helping disperse alcohol from the body. In addition, the vitamins and minerals such as calcium, phosphorus and iron contained in water radish help aid digestion and *qi* flow, and improve eyesight.

Chinese Yam

Chinese yam is very nutritious, and the most important nutritional component is diosgenin, which is known as natural DHEA (dehydroepiandrosterone). These ingredients can help the body synthesize various hormones, promote the metabolism of the skin's epidermal cells, improve the skin's hydration, and also help improve the overall constitution.

Chinese yam is rich in cellulose, choline and other ingredients which supply a large amount of the mucoprotein needed by the human body. This mucoprotein is a mixture of polysaccharides and protein, and has a great effect on the health of the human body. Mucoprotein helps prevent fat build-up in the cardiovascular system, maintaining the elasticity of blood vessels and preventing premature atherosclerosis. At the same time, mucoprotein also reduces the accumulation of subcutaneous fat, protecting against weight gain. Moreover, when combined with inorganic salts, this mucopolysaccharide can also form bone, and make cartilage elastic which helps prevent fractures.

People who plan to take supplements in winter should also make sure they eat some yam, to help absorption. Chinese yam is a medicine that helps invigorate the spleen-stomach and replenish *qi*. It is recommended for consumption before other supplements by people with a weak spleen and stomach.

Medicinal Food Recipes

Traditional Chinese medicinal recipes offer a wealth of health benefits. Eating in a mindful, health-oriented way can achieve twice the health results with half of the effort. The specific type of medicinal diet that will most benefit an individual varies from person to person. Older or middle-aged people should prioritize medicinal porridges and congees, cakes, soup and so on. Here we recommend some types of porridge most suitable for middle-aged and older people, which have the effects of strengthening the body and improving longevity.

① Astragalus Porridge

Ingredients: 30 g raw astragalus, 50 g rice, a little brown sugar

Method: Cut raw astragalus into slices (or buy astragalus slices), put them into an aluminum pot, add some water, and boil them to make juice. Wash the rice, put it into the pot with astragalus juice, add some water, bring to the boil on high heat, then lower the heat and simmer.

Effects: It helps replenish vital *qi*, strengthens the spleen and stomach, promotes hydration and reduces swelling. Long-term use can prolong life.

② Chinese Wolfberry Congee

Ingredients: 15 g Chinese wolfberry, 50 g rice

Method: Wash the berries and the rice, put them in the pot together, add some water, bring to the boil on high heat, and then simmer them into a congee.

Effects: It tonifies the kidney and blood, nourishes *yin* and improves the vision. This recipe has a certain effect on the prevention and treatment of common cardiovascular diseases and diabetes in middle-aged and elderly people, and also aids treatment of blindness and vision loss.

③ Sesame Congee

Ingredients: 6 g black sesame, 50 g rice, a little honey

Method: Fry the black sesame slightly, and then grind it into powder. Wash the rice, put it in the pot, bring to the boil on high heat and then simmer until it soft. Add the black sesame powder and honey, and continue to cook until the rice becomes congee.

Effects: It hydrates the intestines and relieves constipation, benefiting all five internal organs, and strengthening the muscles and bones. Long-term use has significant anti-aging effects.

④ Chrysanthemum Congee

Ingredients: 15 g chrysanthemum powder, 50 g rice

Method: Remove the stem of the chrysanthemum, then steam and dry it (or, just use pre-dried chrysanthemum). Grind it into fine powder and put aside. Wash the rice, put it into a pot and add some water, bring to the boil on high heat, then simmer on low heat until it's half-cooked. Add the chrysanthemum powder, and continue to boil until it turns to congee.

Effects: It dispels wind-heat, clears liver fire, and lowers blood pressure. It's helpful in the treatment of hypertension, coronary heart disease, headaches and other ailments.

⑤ Walnut Congee

Ingredients: one to five walnuts, 50 g rice

Method: Crush the walnuts and wash the rice, then put both into a pot. Add some water, bring to the boil on high heat, then simmer on low heat until congee is formed.

Effects: It helps improve hair health, invigorates the brain, and increases mental dexterity.

⑥ Ginseng Chicken Roll

Ingredients: six fatty chicken legs, 15 g ginseng

Method: Remove the bones from the chicken legs, then

salt the meat and marinate for ten minutes. Set aside. Rinse the ginseng and cut off the ends and stems, shape it to fit the size of the bone, and stuff it into the chicken leg meat, then wrap with gauze and steam it in the pot for 20 minutes. Remove from the steamer and allow it to cool before serving in slices.

Effects: It helps replenish original *qi*.

5. Winter Lifestyle

In the three winter months, human metabolism slows. As levels of *yin* and *yang* change in nature, the excessive cold can very easily damage the *yang qi* of the human body. As a result, your winter lifestyle should begin with reigning in your *yin* and safeguarding your *yang*.

Sleeping Earlier, and Rising Later

The Yellow Emperor's Classic of Medicine contains a detailed discussion of the laws of living through the four seasons of the year. In spring and summer, sleeping late and getting up early is a way of conforming to the characteristics of spring and summer in nature, which is conducive to the growth of *yang* in the body; sleeping early and rising early in the fall also conforms to the characteristics of the autumn harvest. Sleeping earlier helps us reign in our *yin* essence, and waking up earlier helps the flow of *yang qi*. In winter, going to bed earlier and getting up later helps us conform to the characteristics of nature. We should appropriately reduce our activities at this time of year so as to avoid disturbing our *yang qi* and wasting *yin* essence. Therefore, traditional health science suggests that people go to bed earlier and get up later in winter. This is beneficial to the preservation of *yang qi* and the accumulation of *yin* essence, and is beneficial to health.

Avoiding Four Mistakes

Mistake one: Wearing too much clothes. In the cold winter, the more you wear, the warmer you will not be. The role of clothing is

SECRETS OF HEALTH AND JOY IN ALL SEASONS

to isolate the cold air and keep the body warm. Wearing too many clothes, or clothes that are too thick, will affect the metabolism and blood circulation of the human body and actually make people feel cold. Some people like to wear thick clothes to bed in winter, but this is neither warm nor healthy.

Mistake two: Warming up by eating hot pot. It is very cold in winter, and eating hot, spicy foods such as Chinese-style hot pot can make you feel nice and warm. However, this is a bad idea for some people in winter. People with *yin* or *qi* deficiencies, expressed in symptoms such as a dry mouth and tongue, feverishness in palms and soles, and dry stools should stay away from foods like hot pot.

Mistake three: Keeping the AC on a very high heat. "AC syndrome" as discussed earlier in this book does not only occur in summer, but also in winter. Staying in an air-conditioned room for too long in winter can easily cause a stuffy nose, dry mouth, headaches and other symptoms. Due to the large temperature difference between indoor and outdoor, it is easy to catch a chill when you go outside. Patients with cardiovascular and cerebrovascular diseases should stay away from air conditioning.

Mistake four: Waking up too early for morning exercise. In winter, you should go to bed early and get up late. Doing so helps us nourish both *yang qi* and *yin qi*. For this reason, it is best not to wake up too early to exercise. If the temperature is too low in the morning, it's easy to induce cardiovascular and cerebrovascular problems. It is best to wait until the sun comes out before exercising. In particular, it should be noted that the air quality is extremely poor on foggy days in winter, so it is best to avoid going out at these times.

Foot Baths before Bed

Have you ever had difficulty falling asleep, or found that when you do sleep, it is a restless type of sleep from which you wake very easily? This can be caused by not keeping your feet warm. Traditional Chinese medicine believes that the foot is farthest from the heart and the blood reaches there last. For this reason, sometimes the feet are called "the second heart." There are many acupuncture points on the feet. Doing a good job of foot care will also play a role in overall health care.

Soaking your feet in hot water before going to bed can expand the blood vessels, accelerate blood circulation, improve the nutrition of foot skin and tissues and reduce numbness and soreness in the lower limbs. It may also help relieve or eliminate fatigue, and can play a role in preventing and curing diseases. The feet are the junction of the *yang* and *yin* meridians of the human body, and there are many acupoints here. Soaking the feet is equivalent to stimulating these acupoints, thus promoting the circulation of *qi* and blood. For those who suffer from insomnia, who have varicose veins or who work or study late at night, soaking the feet in hot water every night can relieve symptoms and aid sleep.

The method of foot bath is very particular, however. The correct way to soak your feet is with warm water at about 40℃. You also need to rub your feet with your hands constantly, for 15 to 30 minutes. For people with a cold constitution, adding some mugwort leaves to the water can make you feel refreshed and relaxed, and prevent frostbite. However, it is worth pointing out that the water should not be too hot, as this can cause excessive expansion of blood vessels and excessive flow of blood to the lower limbs, resulting in insufficient blood supply to other important organs, leaving you prone to cardio-cerebrovascular problems. Do not spend too long soaking the feet, so as not to increase the burden on the heart; and do not soak your feet within half an hour after eating. Cardiovascular patients should be careful when they soak their feet. In case of dizziness, palpitation, shortness of breath, etc., they should stop soaking their feet immediately.

Keeping Warm

The most important thing that keeps you warm in winter is, clearly, your clothing, but specifics vary from person to person.

Research shows that when the surface temperature of clothes is about 0 ℃, keeping the temperature between the inner layer of clothes and the skin at 32 to 33 ℃ creates an optimum microclimate around the skin of the human body. This effectively buffers the attack of external cold weather and helps maintain a constant temperature.

As for the elderly, due to the decline of their physiological function and low metabolic level, winter clothes should be light and warm. Young people have strong metabolisms and stronger self-regulation functions, so should not wear anything too thick. Infants and young children are slightly different. On the one hand, they are delicate and have poor ability to regulate their body temperature, so more attention should be paid to keeping them warm. On the other hand, human metabolism is exuberant when one is young, and children should not be covered with too many clothes as this can make them sweat too much and affect their health.

Protecting the Nose

Traditional Chinese medicine believes that the nose is the gateway to the lungs, which is the portal of the respiratory system and the main pathway through which pathogens can enter the body. Therefore, the nose reflects the health of the lungs and any abnormalities there should be paid attention to. Nasal congestion, a runny nose, poor sense of smell, flaring of nares, coughing and dyspnea or any other abnormal phenomena can be used as the diagnostic basis for a series of pathologies in the respiratory tract and lungs. Especially in the cold weather, the adhesion of pathogenic bacteria and the stimulation of cold air will lead to the susceptibility of the nasal mucosa, often causing asthma, chronic bronchitis, pulmonary heart disease and other cardiorespiratory diseases. Making sure we are protecting the nose and other respiratory organs in winter can not only prevent colds, but also prevent respiratory diseases and heart and lung infections.

Moisturizing

When it's very cold outside in winter, the dry and cold climate can cause the blood vessels in the skin layer of the human body to contract to reduce the loss of heat. However, this also causes the blood circulation in the skin layer to slow down and the function of sebaceous glands and sweat glands to reduce, resulting in a large reduction in the moisture and fat content of the skin surface. When combined with the cold wind blowing, the skin's resistance will be greatly weakened. Therefore, it's very easy for the skin in winter to become dry, sensitive, and chapped. In terms of diet, it's a good idea to eat plenty of sticky foods, such as honey, sea cucumber, agaric, juicy pears, and so on. This improves the levels of colloid in the blood and can strengthen the preservation of water in cells. The following methods can also be used for skin care in winter.

Dry skin types: Dry skin is extra sensitive in winter and can be maintained according to the following methods.

Method One: Mash half a banana into paste, mix it with a spoonful of honey, smear it on the face, when the mask turns dry, wash with cold water and dry with a towel.

Method Two: Wash your face with two tablespoons of milk, and wash with cold water after drying.

Method Three: Add a few drops of olive oil to some turmeric powder, mix well, smear on the face, and wash it with warm water after drying.

Neutral skin types: Try the following methods to protect neutral skin.

Method One: Add a few drops of orange juice or tomato juice into a moisturizing cream, mix well and smear on the face to make the skin smooth.

Method Two: When eating apples, don't throw away the skin. Apple skin is a good skin cleanser, and you can use it to wipe your face.

Method Three: Take a piece of papaya, cut it and rub gently on the face to make skin soft and bright.

Oily skin types: The biggest feature of oily skin is that sebum secretion is strong, so special attention should be paid to oil removal. You can try the following three methods.

Method One: Take two to three almonds, grind them, mix them with a spoonful of honey, and smear them on the face. Massage for 10 to 15 minutes, and then wash with cold water. This method can remove excess oil and make the skin soft and bright.

Method Two: Add a spoonful of salt to bottled water, and spray the face with this salt water several times a day. After a few days, the skin will have a great change.

Method Three: Use a nourishing face cream to massage the face every morning.

Don't "Hold"

When winter comes, health care should also be changed in due time. In winter, "holding" is a bad idea and can easily make you sick.

Not going to the bathroom: The cold climate in winter means that some people are reluctant to go to bathroom. However, holding your urine and stools at times like this is very harmful to the body. Holding urine for a long time will make the urine in the bladder accumulate. If urine, which contains bacteria and toxic substances, is not discharged in time, it can easily cause cystitis, urethritis, painful urination, hematuria or enuresis and other diseases. In severe cases, urinary tract infections can also spread to the kidneys, causing pyelonephritis, and even affecting renal function. Research shows that the incidence rate of prostate diseases and bladder cancer is significantly higher in people who often hold their urine. If stools are not discharged in time, then water will be absorbed by the intestine again, resulting in dry stools which are more difficult to pass. If toxins in stool accumulate in the body for a long time, and harmful substances are absorbed by the intestines, it will lead to symptoms such as listlessness, dizziness and weakness, and loss of appetite. In addition, if this continues for a long time, it can even damage your gut biome, resulting in a series of anorectal diseases such as constipation, anal fissure, hemorrhoids, and even intestinal cancer.

Not ejaculating or having sex: Traditional Chinese medicine believes that the key to health preservation in winter is to "preserve," so some people have a one-sided view that we should not have sex in winter or ejaculate even if we have sex. In fact, this practice is very harmful to our health. If semen accumulates in the seminal vesicle for too long, when it is finally discharged, the testicles will be subjected to "high pressure" which can lead to the loss of spermatogenic ability. Over time, it can even lead to testicular atrophy, loss of sexual function, and physical pain. In addition, if you deliberately refrain from ejaculating for a long time, it can lead to chronic prostatitis and other diseases. Ejaculation is a necessary physiological process of the human body, and it should not be forcefully repressed. Allowing nature to take its course is the best way.

Not going outside: In the cold weather in winter, many people prefer to stay at home, especially the elderly or those who are less physically strong. Since there is less sunshine in winter, the body's biological clock can't adapt to the change of the short sunshine time, and if you stay at home for a long time, it can disrupt your circadian rhythms and lead to endocrine disorders. These can lead to you becoming irritable, melancholy and easily fatigued or distracted. Staying indoors for too long can also lead to a decline in resistance, so rather than keeping you healthy, on the contrary, it actually makes it easier to get sick. Therefore, try not to stay at home for lengthy periods during the winter. It is best to spend plenty of time outside, going to places with lots of fresh air and space for walking, running, practicing Tai Chi, and dancing, which can all help to mobilize your emotions and relieve depression.

6. Emotional Health in Winter

In winter, the cold is the main factor. As far as the human body is concerned, the cold can be reflected in both physical coldness and psychological coldness, or depression of emotions. The cold winter winds, dense clouds, withered vegetation, and withered things often make people feel sad and unhappy. In addition, the days are short and the nights are long, and there is significantly less sunlight. Under these conditions, the brain's pineal gland loses some of the signals it relies on from the sun, and melatonin is secreted in larger quantities, which can make people feel gloomy, depressed and lethargic in their spirit. This kind of emotional disorder that occurs in winter and is related to seasons is sometimes called "seasonal depression," or being emotionally "cold." Below are some methods for dispelling seasonal bad moods.

Getting More Sunlight
Sunlight disperses fog and mist, and also reduces the secretion of melatonin. It is a rare and valuable nutrient. In winter, finding time to put yourself in the sun's rays can really improve the mood, leaving people's spirited, refreshed, happy and relaxed.

Moving More
Sports such as power walking, running, aerobics dancing, Tai Chi, swimming and so on can promote human metabolism, blood circulation and brain excitement. Constant exercise keeps energy levels high, and is an effective means to resolve bad moods.

Listening to Music
Listening to music not only raises people's spirits, but also improves mood, especially elegant and beautiful light music. These songs can directly affect the structure of the brain and brain stem, producing calming, stabilizing, exciting and emotion-regulating effects.

Eating Bananas
Bananas contain a substance that can make the brain produce thrombocytin, which regulates the endocrine system. This helps reduce the secretion of hormones that have adverse effects on the mood, making people feel calmer, happier and more at ease.

Citrus Fragrances

Citrus fruits are not only gorgeous in color, but also fragrant and refreshing. The oils and other aromatic substances contained in them can affect the brain through the nose, and help regulate people's mental activities and emotions.

Brushing the Hair

Every day, combing your hair consciously with a comb or your fingers and massaging your head will help improve blood circulation to the brain, and generates good stimulation of the brain cells. This small act can help keep you in a good mental state, and maintain a stable mood.

7. Physiotherapy and Health in Winter

Traditional Chinese medicine believes that the correspondence between heaven and man is the basic principle of human health preservation, which means that there is an inherent relationship between the human body and nature. In the winter, when it is very cold, we should therefore adjust to the balance of the *qi* of heaven and earth through appropriate physical therapy, enhancing our immune ability and promoting metabolism. Proper massage of relevant acupoints can clear the meridians, promote blood circulation, remove blood stasis, stimulate *yang qi*, promote metabolism and improve blood circulation.

Massaging the Qihai Acupoint

The Qihai acupoint is located in the lower abdomen of the human body, 1.5 cun down from the navel. Massaging the Qihai acupoint has the effect of nourishing vital energy, tonifying the kidney and essence, restoring *yang* and prolonging life.

Massaging the Guanyuan Acupoint

The Guanyuan acupoint is located 3 cun below the navel, on the midline. Massaging the Guanyuan acupoint can replenish *yang*

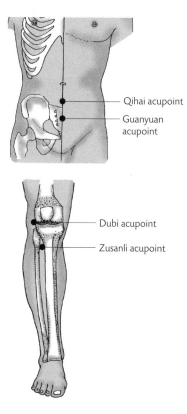

Qihai acupoint

Guanyuan acupoint

Dubi acupoint

Zusanli acupoint

qi, and is effective for relieving neurasthenia, insomnia, cold hands and feet, etc.

Massaging the Zusanli Acupoint

The Zusanli acupoint is located 3 cun below the Dubi acupoint, or about one finger width from the outside of the shin of the lower legs. Massaging this point can expand the microvessels of fingers and toes, increase blood circulation, warm the extremities, improve the immune function of the body, enhance disease resistance, and help prevent and treat stomach disease, abdominal pain, diarrhea, hypertension, anemia, lower limb paralysis and arthritis.

Foot Massage

Nowadays, there are many activities to do at nighttime, and staying up late has become the norm. However, this is an unhealthy lifestyle, and has great hidden dangers to health. Often staying up late leads to hyperactivity of fire due to *yin* deficiency and other problematic symptoms. In addition, due to the cold and dry climate in winter, people often feel drawn to eating hot-natured foods. This however is likely to aggravate inflammation. Instead, foot massage therapy can be very helpful for relieving symptoms. One easy method for massaging the many acupoints on the feet is to walk barefoot for five to ten minutes on an uneven cobblestone pavement (or buy a plastic foot massage mat to use at home). Do this half an hour before going to bed every day.

Appendix
Traditional Chinese Medicine Terms

Terms	Explanations
ascending and dredging	Liver governs ascending and dredging: This phrase refers to the idea that the human liver regulates the rise (ascending) and release (dredging) of *qi* in the body. The liver thus plays an important role in the smooth flow of *qi* throughout the body.
astringent	A medicinal taste that helps restrain, stop, block or slow something.
belt channel	The belt channel is one of the eight extra meridians of the human body. It runs horizontally around the waist and abdomen, circling the body.
clear fluid	Part of the body fluid, which is a clear and thin neutral substance with high fluidity. It is mainly distributed on the surface of the skin, muscles, and pores, and infiltrates the blood vessels, playing a moisturizing role.
clear *yang*	Soft and lucid *yang qi* that rises gently.
clearing heat and promoting diuresis	The treatment method for dampness-heat amassment syndrome using a medicinal recipe with heat clearing and dampness promoting effects.
clearing heat and removing toxicity	A treatment method for diseases such as excessive heat, fire/heat toxins, swelling, and boils. It uses formulas and medicines with the effects of clearing heat pathogens and toxins.
cold	The medicinal properties with functions such as clearing heat, purging fire, detoxifying, and cooling the blood.
concentrating on the elixir field	When practicing *qigong*, this refers to the focus of the mind on the Guanyuan acupoint 3 cun below the navel. Elixir field: The name of a human body part located at the Guanyuan acupoint 3 cun below the navel.
consumptive disease	A disease characterized by deficiency and decline, featuring a shortage of *yin* and *yang*, *qi* and blood, and consumptive disease in *fu* and *zang* organs.

Terms	Explanations
cool	A type of medicine properties which helps with clearing hectic heat.
cooling the blood for hemostasis	It refers to the treatment of syndrome of stirring blood due to intense heat, with the effect of clearing heat, cooling the blood, and stopping bleeding.
cooling the blood for calming endogenous wind	A treatment method for stirring wind syndrome due to blood heat, using a formula with the effects of clearing heat, cooling the blood, calming chills and relieving spasms.
dampness pathogen	Pathogenic *qi* with characteristics such as easily obstructing *qi*, turbidity, viscosity, and tendency to descend.
defensive *qi*	*Qi* that is dispersed outside the meridians and helps safeguard human health.
deficient and cold pathogens	Deficient pathogens refer to: ① the body is deficient and thus receptive to pathogens; ② pathogens transmitted from mother (primary) organ to child (secondary) organ. Cold pathogens refer to an evil energy characterized by coldness, stagnation, and contraction.
dispersing stagnated liver *qi*	Relieving the symptoms caused by liver *qi* stagnation.
dryness pathogen	A pathogen that is prone to damage the lungs and body fluids.
eliminating dampness and facilitating diuresis	Anything that helps expel dampness pathogens via the urine.
essence	All tangible and trace substances in the human body, including *qi*, blood, fluid, and nutrients from food and water.
essential *qi*	The general term for human essence and *qi*.
external assault by wind-cold	Wind-cold pathogens invading the human body from the outside.
five flavors	A general (not literal; there are more than five) term for the different functional types of Chinese medicine: pungent, sweet, sour, bitter, salty, tasteless, astringent, etc.
flaring up of deficient fire	Pathological changes such as dryness of the throat, sore throat, and sores in the mouth and tongue due to *yin* deficiency, where internal water does not regulate internal fire, thus leading to rising up of the deficient fire.

Terms	Explanations
freeing strangury	A type of treatment method using medicines that clear heat and promote diuresis so as to clear the dampness and heat in lower *jiao* and eliminate bodily stones.
heart fire	Excessive *yang qi* in the heart is called heart fire. Moderate *yang qi* in the heart can maintain human vitality, while excessive *yang qi* can be harmful.
heart *yin*	The *yin qi* of the heart, in contrast to the *yang qi* of the heart, is a tranquil, defensive, and nourishing presence, and can also restrain excessive *yang* heat.
heat syndrome	It is caused by heat pathogens or excessive *yang qi* invading the body. Characterized by a higher body temperature, irritability, redness of the face and eyes, dry lips or a dry throat, excessive thirst, cravings for cold drinks, constipation, less and dark colored urine, and a red tongue with yellow coating.
hot	The medicinal properties of nourishing *yang qi* and dispelling pathogenic cold factors.
hyperactivity of fire due to *yin* deficiency	It refers to the pathology where *yin* does not balance *yang*, and *yang* is relatively hyperactive, resulting in the thriving of deficient fire. This can manifest as symptoms such as irritability, redness in the cheeks, and excessive libido.
internal retention of damp-heat	This refers to the accumulation of dampness and heat in the spleen, stomach, and liver and gallbladder of the middle *jiao*. Dampness is a pathogen related to heaviness, turbidity, and stickiness, all of which can affect the circulation of *qi*. If internal retention of dampness is combined with heat pathogens, the heat is difficult to clear due to the obstruction of the dampness, and the dampness is steamed by heat, making the damage to *yang qi* more severe.
internal wind caused by heat accumulation	The wind here refers to the internal wind (which must be distinguished from the external wind, one of the six climatic exopathogens), which means involuntary and uncontrollable movements and mental abnormalities in the body. These are mostly caused by excessive stagnation of heat and loss of *yin* fluid in the body.
invigorating the spleen-stomach and replenishing *qi*	A treatment method for spleen and stomach *qi* deficiency syndrome using formulas and medicines that tonify *qi*, strengthening the spleen and the stomach.

Terms	Explanations
invigorating the spleen and dispersing stagnated liver-energy	A method for treating spleen dysfunction caused by liver *qi* stagnation.
Jueyin Pericardium Meridian of Hand (PC)	The Jueyin Pericardium Meridian of Hand (PC) is one of the 12 meridians of the human body, along with the Taiyin Lung Meridian of Hand (LU), Shaoyang Gallbladder Meridian of Foot (GB), Shaoyin Heart Meridian of Hand (HT), Yangming Large Intestine Meridian of Hand (LI), Shaoyang *San Jiao* Meridian of Hand (TE), Taiyang Small Intestine Meridian of Hand (SI), Yangming Stomach Meridian of Foot (ST), Taiyang Bladder Meridian of Foot (BL), Taiyin Spleen Meridian of Foot (SP), Jueyin Liver Meridian of Foot (LR), and Shaoyin Kidney Meridian of Foot (KI). Meridian: Pathways in the body through which *qi* and blood flow. They connect the organs, and are a channel of communication both internally and externally, running both up and down.
kidney *qi*	The *qi* generated by kidney essence. It is manifested as kidney's functional activities of promoting the growth, development, and reproduction, etc.
kidney *yang*	*Yang qi* in the kidney, which is the fundamental source of *yang qi* throughout the human body.
liver controlling conveyance and dispersion	A description of the idea that the liver has the physiological function of maintaining the smooth flow of *qi* throughout the body, and preventing stagnation.
liver fire	Liver fire is the *yang qi* expression of liver hyperactivity. Moderate *yang qi* in the liver can help maintain human vitality, however excessive *yang qi* can be harmful to health.
liver *qi*	The essence and *qi* of the liver, in contrast to liver blood, are manifested as the functional activities of the liver in regulating blood circulation and storage. Liver *qi* also refers to the *qi* movement of the liver.
liver wind	It describes abnormal liver *qi*, or disorders caused by abnormal liver *qi*.
liver *yang*	*Yang qi* of the liver. Liver *yang* is responsible for ascending and dredging *qi*.
liver *yin*	The *yin qi* of the liver, in contrast to liver *yang*. The nourishing, tranquil, and gentle side of the liver, and can help regulate excessive liver *yang*.

Terms	Explanations
lower *jiao*	The lower part of the *san jiao* refers to the lower abdominal cavity from the outlet of the stomach to the lower part of the groin. It can differentiate between clear and turbidity, infiltrate the bladder, excrete waste materials, and regulate the downward movement of *qi*. *San jiao*: The collective term for the upper, middle, and lower *jiao*, which is not only a division concept of the body cavity, but also a functional concept, as one of the six *fu* organs.
lung governing regulation of water passages	It describes the process of dispersing, purifying and descending of the lung *qi*, creating a dredging and regulating effect on the distribution, movement, and excretion of water and fluid in the body.
lung governing the skin and hair	Human skin and hair rely on the essence and *qi* of the lungs for nourishment and warmth, and the dissipation of *qi* of the skin and the opening and closing of sweat pores are closely related to the lung's function of governing diffusion.
lung *qi*	It refers to the essence *qi* of the lungs.
nourishing the blood and promoting granulation	A treatment method that uses medicines or other therapies with blood nourishing effects, helping promote any type of bodily growth, accelerate the healing of sores, or treat the later stages of sores due to insufficient *yin* blood.
nourishing *yin*	Medicines with a sweet taste and a cool nature, which have the effect of nourishing *yin* fluid, are used to treat *yin* deficiency syndrome. *Yin* deficiency syndrome refers to a lack of *yin* essence and *yin* fluid, characterized by being underweight, having spells of dizziness and tinnitus, a dry mouth and throat, constipation or dark colored urine. Sufferers may also have symptoms such as hot flashes in the afternoon, redness in the cheeks, night sweats, or a reddish tongue with little or no coating.
nourishing *yin* and reinforcing *yang*	Nourishing *yin* means nourishing *yin* fluid. Reinforcing *yang* refers to helping the human body consolidate *yang qi* within the body.
nutrient *qi* and defensive *qi*	These two types of *qi* come from the same source, and are both generated by the essence of nutrients from foods and drinks. Nutrient *qi* is found inside the meridians, while defensive *qi* is found outside them.
nutrient-blood	Nutrients that reside within the meridians and blood vessels to maintain human bodily functions.

Terms	Explanations
original *qi* (*yuan qi*)	Humans are born with original *qi* stored in the kidneys. This *qi* relies on acquired essence to replenish and maintain itself, and is the basic material and driving force of human life and activity. Its main function is to promote bodily growth and development, as well as warming and stimulating the physiological functions of organs, meridians and other tissues and organs.
original *qi* of the lower *jiao*	The vital *qi* of the lower *jiao*. Vital *qi*: The fundamental *qi* that can transform into various other *qi* sources in the human body.
pathogenic *qi*	A collective term for various pathogenic factors.
pungent	A type of medicine taste that can disperse, stimulate, and moisturize.
qi movement	The movement of *qi* takes the basic forms of ascending, descending, exiting, and entering.
qi transformation	Various changes generated through the movement of *qi*, manifested in the metabolism and mutual transformation of essence, *qi*, blood, and clear fluid.
relieving superficies	It refers to the treatment of illness that has not attached to the vital organs of the human body.
removing liver fire for improving eyesight	A treatment method for eye disease caused by internal heat, using the prescription which clears liver fire, detoxifies and thus improving the eyesight.
resolving superficies syndrome with pungent and cool natured drugs	Treatment for wind-heat superficies syndrome, using medicines that are pungent and cool in nature, which have the effect of dispersing wind and dissipating heat.
seven emotions	The general term for human emotions, including joy, anger, worry, thoughtfulness, sadness, fear and shock. Each is a different reaction made by the human body to objective things or phenomena.
six climatic exopathogens	Referring to the six exogenous pathogenic factors: wind, coldness, summer-heat, dampness (humidity), dryness, and fire (heat).
sour	A type of medicine taste which helps absorption, and has astringent properties.

Terms	Explanations
spirit	In TCM theory, the term "spirit" is an abstract concept. In the broad sense, it encompasses the outward activities of life and refers to the comprehensive whole. This includes the vitality of the body, appearance, complexion, expression of the eyes, speech, and responsiveness. In a narrow sense, spirit is a collective term for cognition, consciousness, and other mental activities.
spleen *qi*	The essence and *qi* of the spleen, which are manifested as the functional activities of the spleen in transporting and transforming the nutrient of food and water and regulating blood. Spleen *qi* also refers to the material basis of physiological function of the spleen.
spleen *yang*	The *yang qi* of the spleen, in contrast to spleen *yin*, has warming, promoting, and ascending properties.
summer-heat pathogen	It refers to a type of pathogenic *qi* found after the Summer Solstice and before the Beginning of Autumn, characterized by being ascending and dispersive.
sweet	A type of medicine taste that can nourish, soothe, and harmonize.
tasteless	A taste of medicine that can reduce dampness or is diuretic.
the intercourse between the heart and kidney	There is a harmonious and balanced relationship between the heart and kidneys. The heart is located in the upper *jiao*, which is associated with fire; The kidney is in the lower *jiao*, and is associated with water. Descending heart fire to the kidneys can help the kidney's water keep warm; ascending kidney water benefits the heart, nourishes the heart *yin*, restricts heart *yang*, and prevents the heart *yang* from becoming excessive.
the liver-eye connection	The meridian of the liver is connected with the visual system, and visual function depends on the conveyance and dispersion of liver *qi* and the nutrition of liver blood. The physiological and pathological conditions of the liver are thus reflected in the eyes.
vital gate	The origin of human *qi* energy and the foundation of life.
vital *qi*	A general term for the normal functional activities of the human body, that is, various bodily functions that maintain health, such as self-regulation, environmental adaptability, resistance to pathogens, the immune system, and natural rehabilitation and self-healing.
warm	The medicinal properties of dispersing external cold, warming the stomach, and promoting the circulation of *qi* and blood.

Terms	Explanations
warming the spleen and stomach	A therapy that warms the spleen and stomach.
wind pathogen	A pathogenic factor caused by cold air and characterized by rapid onset and frequent changes; pain exhibiting a migratory nature that worsens when exposed to cold air; and usually causing complaints in the upper body.
wind-heat	The pathology combining wind and heat, clinically manifested as severe fever, mild aversion to cold, coughing, and feelings of thirst.
yang deficiency	A relative lack of *yang* substances and functions in the body, which can disrupt the internal balance of *yin* and *yang*, leading to a phenomenon of weak *yang* and strong *yin* functions in the body.
yang pathogen	Pathogens with *yang* attributes.
yang qi	*Yang qi*: The positive energies of material things and their movements, such as outward appearance, upward movement, exuberance, lightness, and functionality. It is the opposite of *yin qi*. *Yin qi*: The side of a material thing or movement that has internal, downward, inhibitory, or turbid (sometimes referred to as "negative") attributes.
yin deficiency	A relative lack of negative substances and energy in the human body, which can disrupt the balance of *yin* and *yang*, leading to a phenomenon of weak *yin* and strong *yang* functions in the body.
yin deficiency and internal heat	A disease, also known as fever due to *yin* deficiency. It refers to the fever caused by a deficiency of *yin* fluid in the body and the inability of water elements to balance fire elements in the body.
yin pathogen	Pathogens with *yin* attributes.
yuan-primary point	Located below the elbow and knee joints of the limbs, these are specific acupoints for the passage and retention of original *qi* of organs.